NURSING SERIES

Humor in Health Care:
The Laughter Prescription

2nd Edition

**WESTERN®
SCHOOLS**

By
Enid A. Schwartz, RN, MS, MC, PhD

20 contact hours will be awarded upon successful completion of this course.

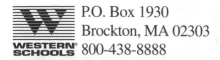

P.O. Box 1930
Brockton, MA 02303
800-438-8888

ABOUT THE AUTHOR

Enid A. Schwartz, RN, MS, MC, PhD, is an instructor in nursing, behavioral health, and psychology. She taught nursing at Cochise College for 17 years, including a course on loss, grief, and dying, which she taught for 11 years on campus and 3 years online. She currently teaches nursing in the classroom for University of Phoenix and online for Grand Canyon University. Dr. Schwartz has presented national workshops on end-of-life issues and care of the dying. She has also taught about humor in health care, aging issues, and Alzheimer's disease for organizations in her community. Dr. Schwartz has several professional publications. She is also a certified laughter leader (CLL) and does laughter workshops in the community. She completed her CLL with the World Laughter Tour in 2004. Her clinical experience ranges from pediatrics to geriatrics. She received a diploma from Newton-Wellesley School of Nursing, a BSN and an MSN from the University of Arizona, a Masters in Counseling from the University of Phoenix, Southeastern Arizona Campus, and her PhD from Walden University. Her dissertation focused on using humor to cope with breast cancer.

    Enid A. Schwartz has disclosed that she has no significant financial or other conflicts of interest pertaining to this course book.

ABOUT THE SUBJECT MATTER REVIEWER

Karyn Buxman, RN, MSN, CSP, CPAE combined her graduate school research with the one thing that enabled her to get through an entire day without losing her sanity: humor. The result became her master's thesis: "The Development and Implementation of a Humor Room in a Hospital Setting." Now an internationally recognized expert on humor, Ms. Buxman puts her studies to work by delivering energy-charged keynote speeches that entertain, motivate, and educate. She has earned the Certified Speaking Professional designation (CSP) and is one of only 29 women in the world to be inducted into the National Speakers Association Speaker Hall of Fame (Council of Peers Award for Excellence, or CPAE). She received the Lifetime Achievement Award from The Association for Applied and Therapeutic Humor (AATH) and was honored by the University of Missouri as one of the distinguished 2003 Faculty Alumni Award winners. She currently serves as President for AATH and has presented for the International Society for Humor Studies. Ms. Buxman has appeared in journals such as *Woman's Day, Shape,* and *Marie Claire* as well as *AJN, AACN Clinical Issues* and *Journal of Psychosocial Nursing.* She is a frequently sought radio and television guest. She's also a contributing author for *Chicken Soup for the Nurse's Soul,* coauthor of *The Service Prescription: Healthcare the Way It Was Meant to Be,* and publisher of *The Journal of Nursing Jocularity,* (the only humor magazine ever published for healthcare professionals). Karyn Buxman is serious about humor.

    Karyn Buxman has disclosed that she has no significant financial or other conflicts of interest pertaining to this course book.

Nurse Planners: Amy Bernard, MS, BSN, RN-BC and Anne Manton, PhD, RN, PMHNP-BC, FAAN, FAEN

    The planners have disclosed that they have no significant financial or other conflicts of interest pertaining to this course book.

Copy Editor: Liz Schaeffer

Indexer: Sylvia Coates

ISBN: 978-1-57801-404-0

COURSE INSTRUCTIONS
IMPORTANT: Read these instructions *BEFORE* proceeding!

COMPLETING THE FINAL EXAMINATION

Enclosed with your course book you will find a FasTrax® answer sheet. Use this answer sheet to respond to all the final exam questions that appear in this course. If the course has less than 100 questions, leave any remaining answer circles on the FasTrax answer sheet blank.

Be sure to fill in circles completely using **blue or black ink.** The FasTrax grading system will not read pencil. If you make an error, you may use correction fluid (such as White Out) to correct it.

FasTrax answer sheets are preprinted with your name and address and the course title. If you are completing more than one course, be sure to record your answers on the correct corresponding answer sheet.

A PASSING SCORE

The final exam is a multiple choice exam. You must score 70% or better in order to pass this course and receive a certificate of completion. Should you fail to achieve the required score, an additional FasTrax answer sheet will be sent to you so that you may make a second attempt to pass the course. You will be allowed three chances to pass the same course without incurring additional charges. After three failed attempts, your file will be closed.

RECORDING YOUR HOURS

Use the Study Time Log provided in this course book to monitor and record the time it takes to complete this course. Upon completion, tally your total time spent and use this information to respond to the final question of the course evaluation.

COURSE EVALUATIONS

The Course Evaluation provided in this course book is a critical component of the course and must be completed and submitted with your final exam. Responses to evaluation statements should be recorded in the lower right hand corner of the FasTrax answer sheet, in the section marked "Evaluation." Evaluations provide Western Schools with vital feedback regarding courses. Your feedback is important to us; please take a few minutes to complete the evaluation.

To provide additional feedback regarding this course, Western Schools services, or to suggest new course topics, use the space provided on the Important Information form found on the back of the FasTrax instruction sheet included with your course. Return the completed form to Western Schools with your final exam.

SUBMITTING THE COMPLETED FINAL EXAM

For your convenience, Western Schools provides a number of exam grading options. Full instructions and complete grading details are listed on the FasTrax instruction sheet provided with this course. If you are mailing your answer sheet(s) to Western Schools, we recommend you make a copy as a back-up.

COURSE COMPLETION TIME FRAMES AND EXTENSIONS

You have two (2) years from the date of purchase to complete this course. If you are not able to complete the course within 2 years, a six (6) month extension may be purchased. If you have not completed the course within 30 months from the original enrollment date, your file will be closed and no certificate will be issued.

CHANGE OF ADDRESS?

In the event that your address changes prior to completing this course, please call our customer service department at 1-800-618-1670, so that we may update your file.

WESTERN SCHOOLS GUARANTEES YOUR SATISFACTION

If any continuing education course fails to meet your expectations, or if you are not satisfied for any reason, you may return the course materials for an exchange or a refund (less shipping and handling) within 30 days. Software, video, and audio courses must be returned unopened. Textbooks must not be written in or marked up in any other way.

Thank you for using Western Schools to fulfill your continuing education needs!

WESTERN SCHOOLS
P.O. Box 1930
Brockton, MA 02303
800-438-8888
www.westernschools.com

WESTERN SCHOOLS
STUDY TIME LOG

HUMOR IN HEALTH CARE:
THE LAUGHTER PRESCRIPTION

INSTRUCTIONS: Use this log sheet to document the amount of time you spend completing this course. Include the time it takes you to read the instructions, read the course book, take the final examination, and complete the evaluation.

	Time Spent	
Date	**Hours**	**Minutes**
_____	_____	_____
_____	_____	_____
_____	_____	_____
_____	_____	_____
_____	_____	_____
_____	_____	_____
_____	_____	_____
_____	_____	_____
_____	_____	_____
_____	_____	_____
_____	_____	_____
_____	_____	_____
_____	_____	_____
_____	_____	_____
_____	_____	_____

TOTAL* [   ]   [   ]

Hours   **Minutes**

* Please use this total study time to answer the final question of the course evaluation.

WESTERN SCHOOLS
COURSE EVALUATION

HUMOR IN HEALTH CARE:
THE LAUGHTER PRESCRIPTION

INSTRUCTIONS: Using the scale below, please respond to the following evaluation statements. All responses should be recorded in the right-hand column of the FasTrax answer sheet, in the section marked "Evaluation." Be sure to fill in each corresponding answer circle completely using blue or black ink. Leave any remaining answer circles blank.

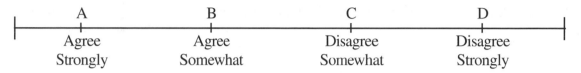

A	B	C	D
Agree	Agree	Disagree	Disagree
Strongly	Somewhat	Somewhat	Strongly

OBJECTIVES: After completing this course, I am able to

1. Discuss the meaning of humor and the theories of humor.
2. Discuss the evolution of humor in health care.
3. Describe how humor develops from infancy to adulthood.
4. Explain how humor can be used in the healthcare setting to benefit patients and their providers.
5. Recognize the psychobiological effects of humor.
6. Discuss the psychosocial effects of humor.
7. Describe how humor can affect the immune system, physiological health, and pain management.
8. Discuss how humor can be helpful to individuals with cancer and other life-threatening illnesses.
9. Discuss the role of humor in crises and disaster situations and discern when healthcare provider intervention is most appropriate.
10. Discuss the effective use of humor in psychiatric settings.
11. Discuss the ways in which humor can be used in educational situations.
12. Describe different types of formal humor programs and the concerns and considerations related to implementing such a program.
13. Discuss ways to engage in humorous interchanges with patients, colleagues, and other healthcare providers.

COURSE CONTENT

14. The course materials were presented in a well organized and clearly written manner.
15. The course content was presented in a fair, unbiased and balanced manner.
16. The course expanded my knowledge and enhanced my skills related to the subject matter.
17. I intend to apply the knowledge and skills I've learned to my nursing practice. (Select the appropriate response below.)

A. Yes   B. Unsure   C. No   D. Not Applicable

continued on next page

ATTESTATION

18. By submitting this answer sheet, I certify that I have read the course materials and personally completed the final examination based on the material presented. Mark "A" for Agree and "B" for Disagree.

COURSE HOURS

19. Choose the response that best represents the total number of clock hours it took to complete this **20 hour** course.

A. More than 22 hours   B. 18–22 hours   C. Less than 18 hours

Note: To provide additional feedback regarding this course, Western Schools services, or to suggest new course topics, use the space provided on the Important Information form found on the back of the FasTrax instruction sheet included with your course.

CONTENTS

FIGURES AND TABLES

PRETEST

1. Begin this course by taking the pretest. Circle the answers to the questions on this page, or write the answers on a separate sheet of paper. Do not log answers to the pretest questions on the FasTrax test sheet included with the course.

2. Compare your answers to the PRETEST KEY located at the end of the Pretest. The pretest key indicates the page where the content of that question is discussed. Make note of the questions you missed, so that you can focus on those areas as you complete the course.

3. Complete the course by reading the chapter and completing the exam questions at the end of the chapter. Answers to these exam questions should be logged on the FasTrax test sheet included with the course.

Note: Choose the one option that BEST answers each question.

1. One important aspect of the definition of humor is that
   a. everyone experiences humor the same way.
   b. humor is individualized.
   c. all humor leads to laughter.
   d. humor is simple to define.

2. An important distinction between humor and laughter is that humor is a cognitive function, whereas laughter is
   a. a release of energy.
   b. a fun experience.
   c. the only response to humor.
   d. a physiological response.

3. The positive effects of humor have been known since
   a. biblical times.
   b. the 13th century.
   c. 1560.
   d. Plato's time.

4. An example of antisocial humor includes
   a. knock-knock jokes.
   b. cultural jokes.
   c. crazy antics.
   d. mispronounced or misused words

5. Children laugh
   a. more than adults.
   b. at everything.
   c. rarely.
   d. only with other children.

6. Release of tension leads to
   a. frustration.
   b. decreased productivity.
   c. increased creativity.
   d. poor problem solving.

7. Nurses need to be careful not to initiate humor with patients
   a. when providing hands-on care.
   b. during the admission procedure.
   c. when the patient is experiencing a stressful event.
   d. when the patient is communicating about a non-stressful situation.

8. As a person begins to read a joke the following part of the brain is activated

    a. pons.
    b. left hemisphere.
    c. right hemisphere.
    d. brain stem.

9. Humor helps to diffuse anger by

    a. bringing people closer together.
    b. releasing pent-up emotions.
    c. increasing awareness to absurdity.
    d. dissolving barriers.

10. Humor works as an effective stress reducer because it

    a. releases endorphins.
    b. suppresses anger.
    c. increases denial.
    d. changes a person's perspective.

11. Using humor as an adjunct to pain therapy

    a. increases the need for pain medication.
    b. decreases endorphin levels.
    c. decreases cytokine levels.
    d. increases the pain threshold.

12. Laughter helps improve

    a. muscle mass.
    b. weight loss.
    c. dancing ability.
    d. respiratory function.

13. People with life-threatening illness find that humor

    a. assists in coping.
    b. depresses them further.
    c. has no effect.
    d. allows them to maintain denial.

14. The use of humor assists victims after a crisis by

    a. allowing the merging of self with the crisis.
    b. decreasing defenses and coping mechanisms.
    c. restricting the survivors' perspectives.
    d. giving perspective on the crisis.

15. In the therapeutic environment, humor is

    a. one way to express caring.
    b. used to mask hostility.
    c. destructive.
    d. anxiety provoking.

16. When used psychotherapeutically, humor can offer the patient

    a. a way of hiding.
    b. insight.
    c. false hope.
    d. assurance.

17. One reason to add humor to the educational process is

    a. laughter is needed to make the material interesting.
    b. humor always aids the learning process.
    c. humor helps to increase motivation.
    d. students like teachers who use humor.

18. Adding humor to the lives of coworkers is as important as sharing humor with patients. One way of doing this appropriately is to

    a. make them the butt of a joke.
    b. place cartoons on the bulletin board.
    c. keep a humor diary.
    d. watch sitcoms during work.

19. The most important element of sharing humor with others is

    a. watching funny movies.

    b. finding the humor within yourself.

    c. thinking of funny everyday situations.

    d. remembering an embarrassing story.

20. One way a person can increase humor awareness is to

    a. keep a humor diary.

    b. participate in a humor study.

    c. watch dramatic movies.

    d. read the personal ads.

PRETEST KEY

1.	B	Chapter 1
2.	D	Chapter 1
3.	A	Chapter 2
4.	B	Chapter 3
5.	A	Chapter 3
6.	C	Chapter 4
7.	C	Chapter 4
8.	B	Chapter 5
9.	B	Chapter 6
10.	D	Chapter 6
11.	D	Chapter 7
12.	D	Chapter 7
13.	A	Chapter 8
14.	D	Chapter 9
15.	A	Chapter 10
16.	B	Chapter 10
17.	C	Chapter 11
18.	B	Chapter 12
19.	B	Chapter 13
20.	A	Chapter 13

INTRODUCTION

The positive effects of humor have been known since biblical times, as noted in Proverbs 17:22 which states, "A merry heart doeth good like a medicine; but a broken spirit drieth the bones." The thirteenth century physician, Henri de Mondeville, believed that laughter assisted in recovery from surgery (Haig, 1988). In 1560, Joubert hypothesized that being joyful and ready to laugh contributed to the health of the mind and the body. He reached this hypothesis after watching three ill people become healthy after laughing at the antics of monkeys (Haig, 1988). In the 1860s Spencer believed that laughter had a tension-relieving effect (Haig, 1988). Within the past 30 years, research on the physiological and psychological effects of humor has increased. Most of this research indicates that humor has a positive influence on the mind and the body.

Klein (1989) states that "humor gives us power and a new perspective" (pg. 3). Studies indicate that it helps us cope with stressful life events, provides strength to get through difficult situations, and offers a different viewpoint on situations (Klein, 1989; Kuiper, Martin, & Olinger, 1993; Lefcourt & Martin, 1983; Nezu, Nezu, & Blissett, 1988; Wiklinski, 1994). Healthcare providers deal with people who are going through stressful life events whenever they come in contact with patients. Having an understanding of how humor can work to decrease tension, improve the viewpoint of a stressful situation, and help cope with life events may give confidence to healthcare providers and encourage them to add humor to their interventions. That is one area of concentration in this program.

Humor has been proven helpful in managing pain. Some of the information on pain management comes from stories shared by those who have employed humor to help with their own pain, such as Norman Cousins' book: *Anatomy of an Illness as Perceived by a Patient*. Some studies looking at humor and pain management indicate a positive correlation (Martin, 2001; Mahoney, Burroughs, & Hieatt, 2001). Because humor seems to have a positive effect on pain management, healthcare providers need to be aware of how it works, and what they might be able to do to help the patient utilize humor as an adjunct to pain medication.

One area of humor research that has received a lot of attention is the effect of humor on the immune system. The following effects have been documented: increases in natural killer cell activity, T-cell activity, immunoglobulins, and some leukocytes (Berk, Felten, Tan, Bittman, & Westengard, 2001). Decreases in the body's production of cortisol after viewing humor films have been reported (Martin, 2001). Increased cortisol levels decreases the bodies immune capabilities. Therefore, the use of humor may increase individuals' protection against certain diseases.

Considering the positive effects of humor shown by research, it is important for healthcare providers to take humor seriously. To that extent, this book was designed to help healthcare providers understand why and how to incorporate humor into the care of patients. The following chapters will look at the history of humor in health care; the effects it has on individuals psychologically, physiologically, and sociologically; how humor develops as we mature; and how to incorporate humor into our own lives and into the lives of others.

Warning # 1: The author of this text takes her humor seriously. This text is meant to educate, not entertain. Anything you find funny is an added bonus.

Warning #2: Don't shoot the messenger. This text is not meant to offend. Humor takes many forms and this text is a demonstration of different types of humor. What might be funny to one person may not be funny to the next person. If you find any portion of this offensive, let that increase your awareness that something else in this text might be offensive to another reader, and be a reminder of why it is important to use humor judiciously.

This continuing education program will examine the holistic effects of humor on the health of individuals. This course will look at the difference between humor and laughter, the development of humor studies, and how humor affects the biological, psychological, and sociological health of individual. The last part of this text will discuss ways in which healthcare providers can incorporate humor into care of individuals and their families. Evidenced-based practice is an important element in health care today. To support the suggestions regarding humor in practice, this text offers discussion of different studies pointing out the efficacy of humor in health care. The study results can be used as evidence to encourage others to incorporate humor into their plan of care. Suggestions for different methods of adding humor as an individual or as a facility are offered.

The target population for this course is any healthcare provider who works with patients, as well as any healthcare provider who wants to improve his or her knowledge of therapeutic humor.

CHAPTER 1

DEFINITIONS AND THEORIES OF HUMOR

CHAPTER OBJECTIVES

After completing this chapter, the reader will be able to discuss the meaning of humor and the theories of humor.

LEARNING OBJECTIVES

After studying this chapter, the learner will be able to

1. define humor.
2. define therapeutic humor.
3. describe the differences between humor and laughter.
4. discuss different theories of humor.

INTRODUCTION

Humor is something that thrives between man's aspirations and his limitations. There is more logic in humor than in anything else. Because, you see, humor is truth.

— Victor Borge

What is humor? That is a question that has not been answered in a way that leads to total agreement. We do know that humor and laughter are universal human experiences, enjoyed by virtually all individuals regardless of culture. Scholars and non-scholars alike have tried to define it. One thing we know is humor and humorous material has many different facets. Each of us has our own view of what is and what is not funny. This chapter will attempt to offer a working definition of humor. Because the text will talk about therapeutic humor and its application to the healthcare environment, therapeutic humor will also be described. To further complicate the issue of humor, there are a number of different theories about what makes humor funny. These theories will be discussed. In some cases, illustrations are included to help explain a particular theory. As you read this chapter, remember that what is funny to one person might be offensive to another. The jokes used in this text are used for illustration of information. If you find the jokes or comments offensive, please remember that someone else might not, but they might find what you think is funny is offensive or a poor illustration.

DEFINITION OF HUMOR

The word *humor* has many definitions. It is a multifaceted response to stimuli. In order to have some understanding of what humor is, it is important to examine how different individuals define it. During this discussion, remember that many disciplines have attempted to define and explain humor.

Philosophers, psychologists, psychoanalysts, anthropologists, sociologists, physiologists, dramatists, playwrights, poets, prose writers, satirists,

1

comedians, and others have attempted to define humor (Robinson, 1991). Ziegler (1998) notes that humor may be looked at as "communication (written, verbal, drawn or otherwise displayed) including teasing, jokes, witticisms, satire, sarcasm, cartoon, puns, clowning which induces (or is intended to induce) amusement, with or without laughing or smiling" (p. 342). Shibles (2002) states that it is a "mistake (and also a joke) to think there is a single definition of humor" (chap. 3, p. 3).

The current word *humor* is derived from two words, the Latin word *umor* and the medieval word *humor,* meaning fluid. Both of these words were medical terms referring to a biological temperament or disposition (Bokun, 1986). One use of the term in this context is humoral theory, the classical theory of health and illness. The humoral theory was based on the four body fluids referred to as *humors:* black bile, yellow bile, phlegm, and blood. Each of these humors was associated with mood: yellow bile (or choler), anger; black bile, melancholy; phlegm, apathy; and blood, confidence (Seaward, 1992). Variations in temperaments and illness were believed to result when the humors were mixed in different quantities. The combination of these body fluids resulted in a person being in "good humor" or "bad humor" (Haig, 1988). Physiologically, humor can be viewed as fluid within the body, such as blood or lymph. Bottari (2000) noted, "What better way to help heal anyone than by getting his/her own body to react to the healing process of engaging the blood and the lymphatic system" (p. 2).

According to *Webster's New World College Dictionary* (2009), humor is "the quality that makes something seem funny, amusing, or ludicrous." Another definition is "the ability to perceive, appreciate, or express what is funny, amusing, or ludicrous." The former refers to the state of something being amusing or absurd. The other refers to an individual's ability to perceive and appreciate something as humorous.

Vera Robinson (1991), one of the first nurses to write about the use of humor in healthcare settings, defines humor as "any communication which is perceived by any of the interacting parties as humorous and leads to laughing, smiling, and (or) a feeling of amusement" (p. 10). Robinson (1991) also views humor as a "cognitive communication leading to an emotional response of amusement, pleasure and mirth, which results in a behavioral physical response of laughter and its counterparts" (p. 10).

Berger (1987) says humor is "not so much a subject as an attitude, a stance, a 'sense' of things that we adopt, that colors the way we function in the universe" (p. 14). Perhaps it is the way humor "colors the way we function" that enables people to use humor for coping with stressful situations.

Humor is a form of communication. Both *Webster's New World College Dictionary* and Robinson's definitions refer to other's perceptions of the message that is given. Each of us may interpret a message differently. For example, how many times have you been in a situation in which someone said something that was not meant to be funny but another person heard the message in such a way that it seemed funny to him or her? Or, how about a message that was meant to be funny, but the receiver either did not understand the humor or was offended by what was said?

Shibles (2002) mentions that humor is an emotion. Emotions cause bodily feelings and actions. Humor results in feelings and actions in a certain context. In a different environment or emotional state of being, the same thing that caused a humor response in one case may cause a different reaction or level of reaction in a different context. Humor allows us to see ourselves and our situations from diverse, different, curious, and extraordinary perspectives.

The Association for Applied and Therapeutic Humor defines *therapeutic humor* as "any intervention that promotes health and wellness by stimulating a playful discovery, expression, or appreciation of the absurdity or incongruity of life's situations. This intervention may enhance health or be used as a complementary treatment of illness to facilitate healing or coping whether physical, emotional, cognitive, social or spiritual" (Association for Applied and Therapeutic Humor, n.d.). This distinction of therapeutic humor is important because it is the basis for the practice of adding humor to the communication between healthcare provider and client. It is also the basis for encouraging others to employ humor in coping with stressors.

The humanistic psychologist Rollo May defined humor as a healthy way of feeling a "distance" between oneself and the problem, a way of standing off and looking at one's problem with perspective (Humor Matters, n.d.). James Thurber stated that "humor is emotional chaos remembered in tranquility" (Humor Matters, n.d., p.1).

Many of the definitions of humor leave out the negative aspects of humor. Although humor can be used to enhance self or relationships, it can also be used in detrimental or injurious ways. Before leaving this discussion, the focus will shift to negative aspects in order to give the reader a broader perspective and to increase awareness that negative humor can hurt the individual producing the humor and/or the person receiving the "humorous" message. The following discussion will look at four dimensions of humor: self-enhancing, self-defeating, affiliative, and aggressive.

Self-enhancing humor. Self-enhancing humor is humor that demonstrates an amused view of life. Author Ashleigh Brilliant (1988) conveys this type of humor in his observations such as "I have so many wonderful qualities, it's easy to overlook my few disgusting habits," (p. 14) and "Many people don't realize my importance immediately, and a surprising number never realize it at all" (p. 91). When employing this type of humor it works as a way of coping and changing a perspective to a more positive view.

This type of humor works as an emotional regulation strategy (Peterson, 2007). This type of humor relates back to Freud's view that humor can work as a defense mechanism and as a way to relieve tension.

Self-defeating humor. This type of humor is used in a self-depreciating manner in order to gain acceptance from others. It might be seen when a person laughs with others, even if the joke involves ridiculing oneself (Peterson, 2007). Comedienne Elayne Boosler is a master of this type of humor, with comments like "I've never been married, but I say I'm divorced so people won't think there's something wrong with me" (Kaufman, 1991, p. 2). Self-defeating humor may be viewed as denial or repression of one's true feelings as a means of gaining approval from others. It is theorized that this type of humor is "positively related to depression and anxiety and negatively related to psychological well-being and self-esteem" (Peterson, 2007, pg. 31).

Affiliative humor. This type of humor may work to increase cohesiveness by creating a positive atmosphere and decreasing conflict. It is humor used to tell jokes and say funny things as a means of getting others to laugh. For cancer patients, this type of humor worked to deflect the attention away from the cancer and allow others to relax with the cancer survivor. Buxman (2000b) cites a piece from an issue of *Journal of Nursing Jocularity:*

> Ann, a home health nurse, met her new patient, Mr. Jones, a quiet man who had a gorgeous head of hair. His chemotherapy had the potential to cause hair loss, and Ann voiced her concern about how he might react if this were to happen. Mr. Jones just smiled and said he could handle it.
>
> The next day, Ann returned for a follow-up visit. Mrs. Jones opened the door, looking quite upset. Mr. Jones sat in the living room,

wearing a hat and scowling. "What's wrong?" asked Ann.

Mr Jones growled, "You said I might lose hair but this is ridiculous!" He pulled off his hat – he was totally bald!

Ann gasped, then noticed Mr. Jones break into a grin. She looked at his wife, who was also smiling – and holding up his toupee! (p. 27)

Aggressive humor. Aggressive style humor works as a way of distancing self from others. It is viewed as positively associated with hostility, anger, and aggression, and negatively related to conscientiousness and relationship satisfaction (Peterson, 2007). For example, one nurse to another: "What's the difference between a nun and a nurse? A nun only has to serve one god" (Buxman, 2000b, p. 38). This type of humor might also be seen in marital relationship when there is a lot of discord.

Bippus (2000) differentiates between *active humor* and *receptive humor.* Active humor occurs when a person engages in different behaviors to induce amusement in others. Such behaviors include verbal comments, physical humor (making faces, pretending to slip and catch themselves, etc.), poking fun, and pranks. Receptive humor involves activities such as laughing or smiling at another's attempt at humor, being a good sport, or making humor-oriented entertainment choices, such as choosing to go watch a comedy.

Looking at the different definitions of humor, it is apparent that there are many thoughts about what humor is. This is one reason why researching humor is difficult. We can measure laughter and the effect it has, but how do we quantify humor? As this text will demonstrate, however humor is defined, it is an important element in our daily functioning and in maintaining our emotional and physical health.

THE DIFFERENCES BETWEEN LAUGHTER AND HUMOR

Most definitions of humor include the element of laughter. However, humor and laughter do not always go hand in hand. It is actually a misconception that *laughter* and *humor* can be used interchangeably. Humor and laughter are qualitatively different (Mahony, 2000; Sultanoff, 2009). Humor is a cognitive response to a stimulus, whereas laughter is a physiological response. Solomon (1996) explains the cognitive process of humor in three steps, beginning with arousal when we hear or see something funny, followed by problem solving, and finally understanding the resolution, or "getting the joke."

Humor and laughter are words we hear about frequently. We know that understanding or appreciating humor is a cognitive process, but then what is the word that describes the emotion felt when we perceive something as funny? Martin (2007) prefers the word "mirth." He defines mirth as the "distinctive emotion that is elicited by the perception of humor" (Martin, 2007, pg. 8). The emotion of mirth may occur with various degrees of intensity, from mild feelings of amusement to high levels of hilarity. It is the emotion of mirth that is attributed to the biochemical changes that will be discussed later in the text. These changes occur in the brain, autonomic nervous system, and endocrine system and involve a variety of molecules, most specifically, neurotransmitters, hormones, opioids, and neuropeptides.

Not everything a person finds humorous results in the behavior we call laughter. Responses to humor may include a twinkling of the eyes, a giggle, a feeling of lightness within, a change in facial expression, or even a groan. One participant in a study by Schwartz (2006) stated that "humor allows the spirit to be free." Laughter may be a response to tickling, surprise, embarrassment, tension, relief after tension, or play.

As previously mentioned, humor is the perception of something being funny. Mirth is the emotion elicited. Laughter is the physiological response to the cognitive understanding of humor and the emotional feeling of mirth. The psychophysiological aspects of humor have been partitioned into three elements:

1. the stimulus (humor);

2. the emotional response (a feeling of mirth); and

3. the physical response (laughter)
(Sultanoff, 2009).

In addition to laughter, other behavioral responses can occur in response to humor. These responses include smirking, smiling, grinning, giggling, and chuckling. When something is perceived as very funny, a person may start laughing and the laughter can become increasingly physical. Have you ever laughed so hard you cried? Can you remember a time you laughed so hard your abdomen or your face hurt?

The trigger of laughter could be a humorous stimuli or the sound of shared laughter. Provine's (2000a) studies indicate that the physical response we call or experience as laughter usually occurs in a social context. That is why laugh tracks are used in sitcoms. Hearing another laugh often triggers laughter in humans. For example, Annette Goodheart, a humor therapist, comes to workshops with her bear, Charlie. She walks out on stage and starts to giggle. Then the giggle turns into laughter. In the audience, one can hear giggles as Goodheart starts her giggling. As Goodheart continues, almost everyone in the audience begins to giggle and laugh. Eventually, for just about every member of the audience, it is hard not to laugh. Goodheart's approach demonstrates that laughter is infectious and the humor stimulus could be the sound of another's laughter rather than a joke or funny incident.

What is it about laughter that makes it contagious? Provine (2000a), who has studied laughter as a behavior, theorizes that the contagious response of humans to laughter suggests that individuals might have some type of neurological trigger that results in the movement of the thorax, larynx, and vocal chords that creates the sound of laughter. He refers to this neurological trigger as the "laugh-detector." This laugh-dector somehow activates the laugh-generator.

HUMOR THEORIES

Humor is multifaceted. It is the lack of a universally accepted definition that makes the study of humor and its effects complicated. The theories that arise because of these multifaceted aspects cover the nature of humor or the purpose of humor. Other theories describe the nature of laughter. Sometimes humor and laughter are used interchangeably. However, as previously noted, the two are not synonymous.

What makes things appear funny or humorous? Multiple theories have been developed to attempt to explain the phenomenon (Haig, 1988; Wilson, 1979), yet the concept remains difficult to define. Wilson (1979) notes that humor, which is everywhere, seems to defy examination. Scholars have been trying to define the essence of humor since the era of Plato and Aristotle (Haig, 1988; Holland, 1982; Wilson, 1979). This attempt continues today.

Haig (1988) examined more than 100 theories about humor and organized them into five theoretical categories: tension-release theories, theories of superiority, theories of social communication, psychoanalytic theories, and incongruity theories. Berger (1987) claims there are three important theories of humor: superiority theory, psychoanalytic theory, and cognitive theory. Harvey (1998) discusses play theory, which is based on a belief that play is an important part of humor. However, according to Holland (1982), none of these theories have reached general acceptance. Table 1-1 provides an overview of humor theories.

TABLE 1-1: OVERVIEW OF HUMOR THEORIES	
Superiority	Laughing at those who make mistakes
Psychoanalytic	A socially accepted way of suppressing unaccepted behavior, such as with sexual jokes
Incongruity	Results of the joke or experience are incongruent
Cognitive	The brain's processing of information that leads to a resolution that produces a sense of amusement
Play	Playfulness that allows the person to see the humorous parts of life or cause laughter in others

Superiority Theory

According to the Greek philosophers Plato and Aristotle, comedy was a way of imitating the worst of man. Some philosophers saw laughter as a weapon to use against evil and a way to help correct the absurdities of society. Using this type of humor presumably gives pleasure from feelings of superiority when we observe those of lower status and contrast their ways with ours. It was believed that people of wisdom should avoid the outbursts of laughter as it deflated others. Whisonant (1998) notes that this theory has fallen out of favor in the last couple of decades. Although it is true that humor can be used as a way to depict the negative in man, this attitude may have hampered the study of humor and the development of humor theories.

This superiority aspect of humor is exemplified by the pleasure that a person takes when someone makes a mistake. The story about the new student nurse who is sent to the supply room by another nurse to get a fallopian tube is an example of humor that leads to feelings of superiority over those who make mistakes.

"When I worked in surgery, the anesthetist sent students looking for fallopian tubes, Eustachian tubes and an occasional "vein caller." After the initiation and a good laugh, the student was officially an insider and got to participate in pulling jokes on the next batch of students…" (Allnurse.com, n.d.)

Superiority can also be seen in situations in which laughter conveys warmth and empathy. This is based on the recognition that the situation did not happen to us, but it could. This aspect of humor can be described as being on a continuum, from laughing at no one, to laughing at someone or others, to laughing with others at man's general failings, to laughing at oneself. Robinson (1991) notes that laughing at oneself "may be the key ingredient in the coping, survival function of humor and laughter" (p. 20).

Three nurses went to heaven, and were awaiting their turn with St. Peter to plead their case to enter the pearly gates.

The first nurse said, "I worked in an emergency room. We tried our best to help patients, even though occasionally we did lose one. I think I deserve to go to heaven." St. Peter looks at her file and admits her to heaven.

The second nurse says, "I worked in an operating room. It's a very high stress environment and we do our best. Sometimes the patients are too sick and we lose them, but overall we try very hard." St. Peter looks at her file and admits her to heaven.

The third nurse says, "I was a case manager for an HMO."

St. Peter looks at her file. He pulls out a calculator and starts punching away at it furiously, constantly going back to the nurse's file. After a few minutes St. Peter looks up, smiles, and says, "Congratulations! You've been admitted to heaven...for five days!"

Note. From Workjoke.com. Used with permission.

Psychoanalytic Theory

In his 1960 translated book *Jokes and Their Relation to the Unconscious,* Freud stated that jokes are a socially acceptable way of satisfying man's need to repress impulses that are not viewed as socially acceptable. He theorized that humor gives pleasure by permitting brief gratification of some hidden or forbidden wish, at the same time reducing the anxiety occurring from the inhibition of the wish. Freud saw humor as a way for adults to think like children and escape the constraints of rationality and logic. This theory defines humor as a socially acceptable way of releasing built-up tension and nervous energy. This theory is also referred to as *relief theory.*

Freud differentiated between what he considered "innocent" and "tendentious" jokes. Tendentious jokes are those that have sexual or aggressive content and the ability to elicit howling laughter. Innocent jokes have less emotional impact and tend to cause a chuckle or less. Sexual humor allows us to disguise sexual aggression and hostility (Berger, 1987) For example, "Why do women fake orgasm? Because men fake foreplay" (*A Prairie Home Companion Pretty Good Joke Book,* 2005, p. 266).

Laughter has been described as a way to release built up energy. Cundall (2007) notes that Herbert Spencer, a biologist and philosopher, felt that people laugh when physical energies build and individuals are not able to channel that energy into "normal outlets." Laughter occurs with a number of events in our lives. We laugh when we are nervous, we laugh at things we find humorous, and we also laugh when we are frightened. Spencer has mentioned that laughter and humor do not always go together as we do not always laugh when we find something humorous, we might just smile.

Cundall (2007) believes both Spencer and Freud's views "utilize the growing strength of physiological and psychological investigation to understand human behavior" (p. 206). Both are aware of the suddenness of humor and they attempt to explain the suddenness through physiological or psychological terms.

Strubbe (2003) mentions that the laughter of relief may have been our ancestors' way of signaling the passing of a life-and-death threat. This relief response is commonly used in the film industry, when tension and suspense build to a crescendo and then an aside or sight gag is interjected to allow a release. In life, relief laughter can allow a person to cope with stressful or dangerous situations.

Relief humor may be experienced in response to "dirty jokes" because these jokes attempt to deal with the tension of sexual inhibitions. This type of humor might be experienced during times of sorrow. The following is an example of relief humor during a funeral. During the funeral preparations for the author's husband, she asked the rabbis officiating to add a little humor because humor was something important to her husband. Her husband, Joe, loved to talk. At the funeral, one of the rabbis shared his first meeting with Joe. He shared how Joe took him on a tour of the area and stated, "And he talked, and he talked, *and* he talked." Giggles could be heard throughout the funeral home because those who knew Joe well could identify with how he talked. The giggles resulted in less tension for the bereaved.

Incongruity Theory

Many theorists claim that incongruity is the main ingredient of humor. According to Leise (1993), this includes "the ability to perceive absurdity in serious situations" (p. 2). Incongruity theory seems to be the most widely accepted theory. This theory encompasses the element of surprise that comes with the conflict of ideas or emotions that results in a burst of laughter. "The punch line generates a surprise, and an incongruous situation leads to laughter or some kind of humorous response" (Berger, 1987, p. 8). For a joke to be understood according to this theory, there is a cognitive process that occurs. The person telling the joke sets up the situation that had an expected outcome. However, the outcome is not what is expected. When the person realizes that the ending is different than expected, he processes this information and "gets the joke." Plato saw the pun as an example of incongruity (Shelly, 2003). Puns become funny when the intellect recognizes incongruous combinations of ideas.

An example of this theory is seen in fractured communication or the misuse of words. For example, a volunteer entered a patient's room wearing oversized plastic eyeglasses with prescription pill bottles taped on each side of the frames. A young patient said, "I like your glasses." "They're her prescription glasses," deadpanned one of the nurses. The following charting examples also illustrate incongruity theory:

*   "Discharge status: Alive, but without permission."
*   "Patient ate whole tray."
*   "By the time she was admitted to the hospital, her rapid heart had stopped, and she was feeling much better."
*   "Patient referred to hospital by private physician with green stools."
*   "Mycostatin vaginal suppositories. Insert daily until exhausted."

Another example of humor that fits within the incongruity theory is seen in a W.C. Fields joke. Someone asked Mr. Fields, "Do you believe in clubs for young people?" Fields replied, "Only when kindness fails."

Cognitive Theory

Cognitive theory is concerned with the way the brain processes information and focuses on the information we categorize as humor (Berger, 1987). From the cognitive perspective, "humor involves a resolution of logical paradoxes and other logical problems" (Berger, 1987, p. 10). Berger refers to

"Could I make 100 copies of this?"

Note. From DansCartoons.com. Used with permission.

this theory as semiotic, or the science of signs. He contends that a comic film, for example, is a series of signs and codes that people interpret to make meaning. How people process this interpretation (cognitive work) is the focus of semiotic analysis that can lead to the response known as humor.

Cognitive theorists view humor as a coping strategy employed to shift perspectives or change the view of a situation or event. Humor is seen to work as a buffer in two different ways. First, by choosing to view the situation in a humorous way, the situation becomes less threatening. Second, using humor can make stressful situations appear less influential.

> Did you hear about the nurse who died and went straight to hell?
>
> It took her two weeks to realize that she wasn't at work anymore!
>
> *Note.* From Workjoke.com. Used with permission.

Interpretation of a Joke by Four Theorists According to Berger

The following analysis is presented as a means of demonstrating how different theorists might interpret the same joke. As the learner reads the joke, it is important to remember that what is funny to one person might be viewed differently by someone else. The joke is not meant to offend, but to demonstrate. Berger (1987) analyzed a joke from the perspective of the first four theories mentioned above. Let's look at this analysis as a way of understanding how humans can process jokes, with the resulting behavioral response of laughter or at least the emotion of mirth. For his analysis, Berger chose the following joke as an example:

A man goes to Miami for a vacation. After 5 days there, he looks in the mirror and notices he has a gorgeous tan all over his body, except where his thong swimsuit covered him. He decides to remedy the situation. The next morning he gets up early, goes to a deserted section of the beach, and starts putting sand all over his body until only his untanned body part is exposed above the sand. Two little old ladies happen to walk by just as he has finished shoveling the sand all over himself. One of the ladies notices him and tells her friend "When I was 20, I was scared to death of them," she says. "When I was 40, I couldn't get enough of them," she continues. "When I was 60, I couldn't get one to come near me. And now they're growing wild on the beach."

A superiority theorist would say that we laugh because we feel superior to the characters in the story. The man is seen as foolish for thinking he must have a tan at any expense. The woman, who thinks that private parts can grow wild on the beach, demonstrates ignorance.

Freud would have a good time with this joke. From his psychoanalytic viewpoint, the humor response from this joke comes from its sexual content. In this case, humor is related to sexuality and, particularly, sexual hunger as it changes with age. The joke not only has a woman who thinks private body parts can grow wild on the beach but also has a man who demonstrates exhibitionist tendencies.

An incongruity theorist would explain that the humor comes from the absurdity that a person would only have that body part sticking out of the sand or that this body part might grow wild on the beach. The punch line is the incongruent part of the joke. In addition, there is something bizarre about someone burying his body and leaving his private parts open to potential public view. Most of the joke sets up the story, or develops the framework. The last line seems incongruent, which leads to laughter.

From the perspective of a cognitive theorist, the joke has a "play frame" that is established by the man's bizarre behavior and desire to tan every part of his body. According to Berger (1987), "this play frame allows us to view the crazy notion of the woman that penises might grow wild on the beach as funny and not to be taken seriously" (pp. 11-12).

Play Theory

Another theory holds that play is an essential part of humor (Harvey, 1998). Play theory purports that "the enjoyment of something laughable comes from the arousal of a playful mood" (Harvey, 1998, p. 43). McGhee (1994) believes that playfulness is an important element in seeing the humorous parts of life. He states that playfulness is "the basic foundation for your sense of humor" (p. 56). Crundall (2007) states, "in order to take many occurrences of humor as humorous, we must be in the proper play environment" (p. 209). McGhee (1994) also states that playfulness leads to increased spontaneity and enjoyment, which allows the mind to process experiences as more humorous than it can when you are serious. If this is true, then adding a sense of playfulness into health care can result in more enjoyment of the professional aspects of health care and improved relationships between all individuals with whom the provider comes in contact.

Have you ever walked into a room and experienced a sense of tension that felt very uncomfortable? Maybe someone just had a fight with someone else, or maybe someone was dying or in a lot of pain. Whatever the problem, the room felt full of negative vibes. If a measure of playfulness, done with sensitivity and respect, was brought into this environment, theoretically it could help lighten the mood. Take the following situation as an example: A doctor's patient is very ill and the doctor does not want to leave the patient for long. He misses his dinner. He is sitting with the patient when the nurse walks in to see if there is anything she can do. The doctor complains of being hungry and asks her to bring him something. Dietary service is closed, and there is nothing on the unit except custard and juice. The doctor desires something more substantial, but none of the units have anything more to offer. The doctor, probably due to hunger, becomes more irritable. The nurse remembers that the humor cart has a rubber chicken. She gets the chicken, puts a blue ribbon around its neck, folds it into a dish, puts a silver cover over it, and brings it to the doctor. His eyes light up when he sees the dish; he takes the cover off and the chicken unfolds. In anger, he says, "What the hell is this?" The nurse looks and says, "I think it is Chicken Cord n' Blue." At that, the doctor starts to laugh, and the nurse and doctor laugh together. She then brings him the custard and juice, which he finishes joyfully.

> Sign on a maternity room door:
> "Push. Push. Push."
>
> *Note.* From RXForSanity.com. Used with permission.

HUMOR'S MANY FORMS

"Humor is essentially an emotional response of mirth in a social context that is elicited by a perception of playful incongruity and is expressed through smiling and laughter" (Martin, 2007). There may be a common basis of humor, but the events, social situations and interpretations that might elicit humor are diverse. As we go through the day, we react to a variety of different forms of humor that are communicated by different means and for different purposes. Also, how an event strikes us might vary depending on what else is occurring in our lives. How often have you been in a situation that was not funny at the time but later, in the retelling of the story, the absurdity of the situation led to a humorous account of events?

Our day may be bombarded by radio hosts' witty comments or jokes and television programs in the forms of sitcoms, blooper shows, stand-up comedy, political satire, and humorous advertisements. We might pick up a newspaper and read the comics, glance at cartoons, or read a humorous report of an event. Perhaps we'll watch a funny movie or read a humorous book. There are any number of situations that might offer humor in any given day.

Most of the humor and laughter experienced arises spontaneously in our natural environment (Martin, 2007). It might occur from watching a cat at play, or chatting with a friend or coworker. Interpersonal humor might happen in a formal or informal situation, and it might happen between lovers, family, friends, doctors, nurses, store clerks or complete strangers standing in line at the grocery store. It is this spontaneous type of humor that is most often experienced in the healthcare arena. It is staff members sharing a laugh about a difficult subject or patient. It is the social worker reaching out in a humorous manner to help the family deal with new situations and changes in life-style. It is the nurse gently encouraging the newly diagnosed diabetic to administer his or her own insulin. It is the connection that occurs with a smile between the healthcare provider and the patient.

SUMMARY

Humor defies a specific definition. It is a response to stimuli that causes positive changes. The change may be one of mood, attitude, hope, or perhaps a connection to others. Humor is a perception (the stimulus); mirth is emotion produced by humor; laughter is a behavioral response. The physical response to humor is sometimes laughter, but laughter and humor are not the same.

As there are multiple definitions of humor, there are also multiple theories of humor. The most popular one among researchers is incongruity theory. However, in reviewing the theories presented, it is possible to see the areas of validity in each of them. Jokes often are funny because of the element of incongruity. There are times when the relief of tension leads to a laugh to lighten the mood or change a perspective. The element of play and recognition that something is meant to be funny incorporates the cognitive process of understanding with the social aspects of response to others. Whatever theory one believes, we know that humor has physical and psychosocial value.

"That's good. Laughter is the
best medicine."

Note. From DansCartoons.com. Used with permission.

EXAM QUESTIONS

CHAPTER 1
Questions 1-9

Note: Choose the one option that BEST answers each question.

1. The definition of humor consists of which of the following properties?

   a. Communication, feelings of amusement, and multifaceted parts

   b. Communication, a specific definition, and feelings of amusement

   c. Communication, mood alteration ability, and negative physical stimuli

   d. Feelings of amusement, mood alteration ability, and exaggerated response

2. An element of humor found in several of the term's definitions is

   a. its ability to cause feelings of amusement.

   b. its mood-altering effect that simulates morphine's effects.

   c. its ability to produce a negative immunological effect.

   d. the sense of superiority it reflects.

3. Any intervention that promotes health and wellness by stimulating a playful discovery, expression, or appreciation of the absurdity or incongruity of life's situations serves as a definition of

   a. inappropriate humor.

   b. dark humor.

   c. therapeutic humor.

   d. spontaneous humor.

4. Laughter is best defined as

   a. an indicator that humor is effective.

   b. the same as humor.

   c. a learned response to humor.

   d. a behavioral response to humor.

5. The difference between humor and laughter is

   a. humor is a perception; laughter is a feeling.

   b. humor causes a feeling of lightness; laughter causes feelings of tension.

   c. humor is a cognitive response; laughter is a physiological response.

   d. humor causes feelings of mirth; laughter is the cause of humor.

6. The psychophysiological response to humor has been divided into three main elements. These elements are

   a. stimulus, perception, and emotional response.

   b. stimulus, emotional response, and physical response.

   c. emotional response, cognitive response, and physical response.

   d. emotional response, receiver of the message, and behavioral response.

7. A student nurse was taking care of a patient who was on bed rest with commode privileges. When the patient asked to go to the bathroom, the student put the commode on the bed for the patient to use. Recognizing how ridiculous this action was, the nursing instructor started to laugh when she heard this story. This form of humor would most likely fall under the humor theory of

    a. superiority.

    b. social communication.

    c. psychoanalytic.

    d. tension release.

8. According to Freud, a tendentious joke would elicit a

    a. giggle.

    b. smile.

    c. smirk.

    d. howl.

9. The element of humor that occurs in reading nurses' notes that contain misused words falls under the theory of

    a. tension release.

    b. superiority.

    c. incongruity.

    d. social communication.

CHAPTER 2

THE HISTORY OF HUMOR IN HEALTH CARE

CHAPTER OBJECTIVE

After completing this chapter, the reader will be able to discuss the evolution of humor in health care.

LEARNING OBJECTIVES

After studying this chapter, the reader will be able to

1. discuss the early recognition of the importance of humor in health maintenance.

2. discuss the history of humor in health care.

3. describe how the use of humor in health care has changed through the years.

INTRODUCTION

Proverbs 17:22, "A merry heart doeth good like a medicine."
– Proverbs 17:22

As noted in Proverb 17:22, quoted above, the knowledge of the importance of humor in medicine has been around since biblical times. There have been times when humor has been considered inappropriate and unprofessional to be used in healthcare settings. There is still some debate about the appropriateness of using humor in psychiatric care. The concept of humor as a therapeutic tool has received varying support from the scientific and healthcare community at different points in his-

tory. This chapter will look at the growth of humor research and how increased knowledge has affected attitudes and use of humor in the helping professions. Thanks to Vera Robinson, there is knowledge of the use of humor in nursing. Little was found in the literature about the actual use of humor in medicine or the mental health sector of health care. Because of the lack of information concerning the use of humor in other healthcare disciplines, a section of this chapter will review the history of humor in the nursing profession.

THE GROWTH OF HUMOR RESEARCH

Knowledge of the benefits of humor has been around for centuries. During the 16th century, Martin Luther employed humor in his pastoral counseling of depressed people (Wells, 2001). He suggested that they surround themselves with friends who could joke and make them laugh rather than isolate themselves.

In the 1860s, the scientist Herbert Spencer noted that laughter had a tension-relieving effect (Haig, 1988). The psychologist, William McDougall stated in 1903 that laughter stimulated the respiratory and cardiac systems, causing a euphoria that broke up the thoughts of pain and sadness (Haig, 1988). This theory has been substantiated to some extent in various studies. In 1923, McDougall made known his belief that humor served as a survival mechanism because it is nature's antidote to depressing and sad events experienced by humans (Leise, 1993).

According to Strubbe (2003), the scientific study of laughter has contributed an expanding body of research. The field is referred to as gelotology, from the Greek *gelos,* meaning "laughter." The first humor research studies occurred in the 1930s (Gibson, 1995). These studies found that the initial effect of laughter is stimulatory. Pulse and respiratory rates increase with laughter and, after laughter subsides, there is a brief relaxation phase.

The study of humor and health had its true beginnings in the 1960s, with the research of Dr. William Fry. Dr. Fry, a psychiatrist and professor emeritus from Stanford Medical School, became interested in humor research through his study of paralinguistics. Paralinguistics involves nonverbal communication forms, such as sobbing and laughing. Fry was also curious about the physiological responses to humor. Using a pulse oximeter, he investigated the change in oxygen saturation after 3 minutes of continuous laughter. He found there was no change. However, he did find that laughter resulted in increased ventilation, increased muscle activity, increased minute volume, and the creation of forceful exhalation that could mobilize secretions.

In 1976, Norman Cousins wrote an article for the New England Journal of Medicine about his experience using humor in dealing with ankylosing spondylitis, a painful and progressive rheumatoid disease that causes inflammation of all joints, particularly the intervertebral disks of the spine. In 1979, Cousins expanded this article into his famous book, *Anatomy of an Illness as Perceived by the Patient.* In this book, Cousins shared how 10 minutes of hearty laughter provided 2 hours of pain-free sleep. The discussion of the effects of humor by Cousins was anecdotal, but it triggered interest in the use of humor as a pain-management strategy. From the experience of this nonmedical person, the study of humor and health really started to grow.

In 1986, Lefcourt and Martin proposed that humor might be a moderator of life stress (Haig, 1988). They produced evidence demonstrating that humor had a moderating effect on mood in normal college students who were experiencing increasing numbers of negative life events. They developed two questionnaires, the Situational Humor Response Questionnaire (SHRQ) and the Coping and Humor Scale (CHS), both of which are still used in many of the quantitative studies conducted on humor today.

The body of knowledge concerning humor continues to grow. Humor science is no longer seen as frivolous or useless thanks to quantitative data demonstrating positive physical and psychological properties. Some universities have added humor studies to their curriculum. When the author of this text started doing research for a dissertation on the use of humor while coping with breast cancer, there were few studies looking at humor and cancer coping. Six years later, the scientific information had increased. A literature search in 1998 revealed two studies specific for cancer and coping. Today there are more than 10 such studies.

PSYCHO-NEUROIMMUNOLOGY

Before the 1960s, common belief was that the mind and the body were separate entities. However, research examining mind-body interactions has shown that our mental state has a significant effect on our physical health and well-being. Specifically, studies indicate a connection between emotional status and the immune and neuroendocrine system.

The field of psychoneuroimmunology (PNI) began in the 1970s. At that time, this new field of study was considered controversial. However, substantial evidence now supports the belief that the mind and body communicate with one another through a bidirectional flow of hormones, cytokines, and neuropeptides (Watkins, 1997). The increased scientific evidence about the mind-body relationship clearly demonstrates that mood, thoughts, emotions, and belief systems can have an impact on the body's basic healing and health mechanisms (McGhee, 2000).

Studies examining PNI and the influence of humor have focused on the hypothalamus-pituitary-adrenal (HPA) axis and the sympathetic nervous system (Berk, Felten, Tan, Bittman, & Westengard, 2001). Berk and colleagues (2001) refer to the type of stress that is modulated by humor as a eustress experience. Eustress is a positive emotional state. The humor studies these researchers conducted looked at the effect of eustress induced by mirthful laughter on cortisol and catecholamines, which are products of both the HPA axis and the sympathetic nervous system. Additionally, Berk and colleagues (2001) have investigated laughter's effect on other hormones, such as growth hormones and prolactin, and the effect of humor on opioid peptides.

McGhee (2000) notes that some people believe that good coping skills help sustain health and well-being. Improving and taking advantage of a sense of humor is a fun way of coping with daily hassles. Mia Smitt (1995), a hospice nurse, comments that "humor is a PNI therapy." She makes this claim based on evidence that humor is beneficial to health because it enhances the immune system. (Berk et al., 1989). It is also a mediator of stress. The physiological effects of humor, including its effects on the immune system, will be explored in more detail in chapter 3.

THE HISTORY OF HUMOR IN HEALTH CARE

Humor has been used in health care since at least the 13th century. Information about humor use in medicine and other areas of health care is sketchy. However, the use of humor in nursing can be followed since at least the time of Florence Nightingale. From accounts presented in notes on the Crimean War and letters written by Nightingale, it is apparent that humor was one way Nightingale dealt with the horrors, filth, and stresses of war. For example, in 1858, Nightingale wrote a letter to the Secretary of War from Scutari, Crimea, describing the filth. She stated, "The vermin might, if they had but unity of purpose, carry off the four miles of beds on their backs and march them into the War Office" (Kelly, 1981, p. 30).

In her "Duties of Probationer" for the first Training School for Nurses in 1860, Nightingale required nurses to be patient, cheerful, and kindly (Kelly, 1981). She appears to have set the tone for restrained use of humor by reminding students to be sober, trustworthy, honest, chaste, and clean in order to prevent a situation in which an "immodest jest" would be spoken in a nurse's presence.

Looking back over the years, it is apparent that the type of humor in and about nursing has changed. Of course, that is also true about humor in general. There is little, if any, record of the use of humor between patient and nurse before the 1960s. That does not mean that humor was not used, but rather that the deliberate use of humor for communication, teaching, or therapeutic intervention was not documented before that time. The humor that can be found before 1960 tends to reflect patients' perceptions about nurses and the care they received (Robinson, 1991). Robinson (1991) notes that this humor tends to reflect four stereotypical images of nurses: the servant or handmaiden, the nurturer, the sex-object, and the old battle-axe. These perceptions of nurses most likely resulted from patients' fears, anxieties, and misconceptions.

Humor about nurses has changed as nursing has become a more respected profession. Nurses are not depicted in negative stereotypes or as sexual objects as often as they were in previous years. As nursing evolved, the ability of nurses to laugh at themselves grew. The first cartoons about nurses for nurses appeared in *RN* magazine in the early 1940s. For the first 6 months of nursing training, a student was considered a probationer, or "Probie." Many of the cartoons of this era made fun of the "Probie." The cartoons that appeared in *RN* commonly involved dumb student incidents, practical jokes, and gallows humor. This type of humor was often vividly remembered and was therapeutic for the nurse.

The use of patient-related humor is less obvious because it was not encouraged in the 1940s. Such humor did exist, however. There were jokes about hospital gowns that did not cover enough and flapped in the breeze, hospital food, bedpans, and "finishing the bath!" (Robinson, 1991). Jokes about these types of situations were the main types of humor up until the 1960s.

In the 1950s and 1960s, cartoons appeared in *RN,* the *American Journal of Nursing (AJN),* and *Medical Economics.* In 1976, Thelma Canarecci compiled her cartoons in *Odds & Ends of Ward Wit. AJN* also printed a "time off" page, which presented information that offered some lighter, sometimes funny or nostalgic material.

Robinson (1991) notes that during the 1960s, "with the advent of community mental health, psychosocial nursing, recognizing and meeting the emotional needs of patients, moving to a focus on health promotion rather than disease, and a humanistic approach to nursing, that we first began to take humor seriously" (p. 11). Articles that looked at humorous topics or discussed issues regarding the use of humor with patients began appearing in nursing magazines. Humor started to become accepted as a therapeutic tool.

In 1965, Vera Robinson began to research how nurses used humor. She explored the history of humor in health care, particularly between nurses and patients. The research began as a grant from the National Institute of Mental Health (NIMH). She later expanded on this research for her doctoral dissertation. The first school she attended attempted to dissuade her from doing her dissertation on humor because it was not considered a professional subject. She subsequently changed universities so that she could continue to pursue her interest in humor and health care. Today, numerous dissertations on humor in nursing are available. These studies cover such issues as the use of humor by cancer patients (Schwartz, 2006; Wiklinski, 1994); humor communication between nurses and residents in a long-term care residence (Lippert, 2001); and the use of humor as a coping mechanism in prisoners of war (Henman, 2001).

Vera Robinson was also the first nurse to publish a text on humor and the health professions. This text, published in 1978, resulted from the work she had done on her dissertation. Her book covers many aspects of humor and health, including the value of humor in health, the use of humor by nurses when interacting with patients, and ways to bring more humor into healthcare settings. At the time Robinson started her dissertation, using humor was seen as unprofessional. In just 15 years, humor had become a scholarly subject that was considered acceptable to research and teach. In the 1980s, nurses began incorporating humor into education, practice, and management (Robinson, 1991).

From 1982 to 1986 Nurses for Laughter (NFL) was organized by approximately 50 nurses for the purpose of promoting the use of humor in nursing and health care. It grew to more than 1,000 nurses but disbanded due to administrative overload (Robinson, 1995, p. 14).

In 1988, a nurse named Alison Crane started the American Association for Therapeutic Humor (AATH) to advance the dissemination of humor in health care. By 2000, the organization had grown and the name was changed to the Association for Applied and Therapeutic Humor to reflect the direction the association had taken. A number of AATH members are nurses who are well known in the therapeutic humor community, such as Patty Wooten, Karyn Buxman, Leslie Gibson, and Mark Darby. Each of these people has worked to further advance the knowledge of the benefits of therapeutic humor.

A Nursing Humor Journal is Born

Until a tragic accident took his life in 1998, Doug Fletcher was the publisher of *the Journal of Nursing Jocularity (JNJ)*. The first issue of *JNJ* was published in spring of 1991. The magazine was published quarterly for nurses and other health professionals and was written, illustrated, edited, and published completely by nurses and other health professionals. The magazine took risks by presenting humor that was sometimes macabre. However, as Fletcher (1991) stated in one of his editorials, "The closer our work is to pain and death, the darker our humor is. [Emergency room] and [intensive care unit] nurses are some of the sickest nurses I know when it comes to humor" (p. 128). The magazine included articles about the therapeutic use of humor; reviews of current books, tapes, and toys related to humor and health care; jokes; satire; stories; and interviews with experts in the area of psychoneuroimmunology. In its seventh year of publication, *JNJ* had more than 35,000 subscribers from all 50 states and Canada (Wooten, 1997).

JNJ reflected the humor of the present-day nurse. There were jokes and stories about managed care. There were jokes about situations in emergency rooms, intensive care units, and other areas. Some of the humor was dark humor that encouraged laughing about death and disfigurement. This type of humor is sometimes referred to as "gallows" humor because it revolves around someone who is facing disgusting or heartbreaking situations. All humor serves a purpose: to help relieve stress and to make the present situation bearable and lighter. In many cases, the grimmer the situation, the darker the humor becomes.

Along with the magazine, *JNJ* sponsored a humor and health workshop every summer from 1991 until Fletcher's death. The workshops were designed to present information about the use of therapeutic humor in health care, and they contained valuable information about the use of humor. The workshops also served as a means for nurses to recognize the effectiveness of humor as a stress-reduction technique because most of the presentations were designed to elicit laughter.

Prior to his death, Fletcher and several other nurses developed a program called *Who's Got the Keys?* This song-and-dance show was a spoof on nursing, its history, and the effects of managed care on nursing and patient care. A video of the show was made and this author has used the video as a humorous and effective means of educating student nurses.

In January 2009, the former vice-president of the *Journal of Nursing Jocularity*, Karyn Buxman, re-launched the magazine, this time as an online publication (www.JournalOfNursingJocularity.com). Many of the former contributing editors returned with the magazine. The focus of the magazine is still entertainment and education, but it now has the capabilities to include media features, such as audio and video clips, interactive polls and surveys, and forums, which were not possible with a paper publication.

The Development of Laughter Clubs

In 1995 Dr. Mandan Kataria, a medical doctor from Mumbai, India was researching information for a journal article on the benefits of laughter. He was amazed at the amount of information demonstrating positive psychological and physiological benefits of laughter and decided to share this knowledge with people in his community. He did this by gathering four other people and starting a laughter club in the park. The five people laughing in the park soon spread to 50 people, and now laughter yoga club numbers have spread to over 6,000 clubs in 60 countries (Laughter Yoga International, n.d.) In the United States, there are laughter yoga clubs in at least 24 states.

In 1998, Steve Wilson, a psychologist who also refers to himself as a "joyologist," had the opportunity to go to India, where he met Dr. Mandan Kataria, the founder and president of Laughter Club International. Wilson, who has studied humor and health, felt there was great potential for adding joy to people's lives by teaching them a systemic routine for laughing without using jokes. Using Dr. Kataria's laughter yoga principles, and with support from his wife and the assistance of Karyn Buxman, a nurse and professional speaker on humor and health, Wilson developed World Laughter Tour (WLT). The slogan for WLT is "Think Globally, Laugh Locally." Since its inception, "WLT has come to be recognized as a significant global influence in the practical applications of laughter and humor for health and world peace" (WLT, n.d., p. 3).

The WLT offers training classes for those interested in becoming a Certified Laughter Leader (CLL). The classes are 2 days of education and laughter. The information covered includes the science of laughter, plus the theory, philosophy and physical aspects of the laughter exercises that are taught. After the training experience, Laughter Leaders are encouraged to start Laughter Clubs. Laughter Clubs exist in various locations, including nursing homes, assisted living facilities, elementary schools, communities, libraries, and colleges. Many CLLs are nurses, but there are also social workers, psychologists, counselors, healthcare staff workers, and even those who work in construction. Anyone interested in teaching others the benefits of laughter by conducting Laughter Clubs are encouraged to participate in the training classes.

Among the published goals of WLT are:

- To bring people of various countries together and promote events that bring everlasting peace through laughter

- To create a membership-based organization for the support of WLT as a self-sustaining organization

- To disseminate accredited training around the world and to develop models for advanced training using traditional educational methods as well as modern technological innovations, such as distance learning

- To develop a cadre of competent, accredited trainers who can train and certify Laughter Leaders

- To promote the adoption of Laughter Clubs in public places that can be free and open to everyone

Nurstoons
by Carl Elbing

HOW COME MY ASSIGNMENT WAS SWITCHED?

IT'S IN THE **PATIENT'S BEST INTEREST** THAT WE MAINTAIN CONTINUITY OF CARE, SO I SHOULD KEEP MY OLD ASSIGNMENT

I DON'T REMEMBER YOU BEING UPSET **LAST WEEK** WHEN THEY GAVE ME YOUR ASSIGNMENT

THAT WAS **COMPLETELY** DIFFERENT!

THAT ASSIGNMENT WAS **HORRIBLE,** THIS ONE IS **EASY**

Note. From Nurstoon.com. Used with permission.

- To promote the adoption of Laughter Clubs in every long-term care facility in the United States, as well as in schools, government offices, and workplaces, as an effective, reputable, professional program, on a fee-for-service basis wherever it is appropriate

- To create a professional association for accredited Laughter Leaders and providers of therapeutic laughter programs to enhance credibility and spread the access to these methods around the world

- To foster international conferences, meetings, and symposia on the therapeutic benefits of laughter and laughter methods to foster research and the sharing of research findings (WLT, n.d.).

SUMMARY

Humor's ability to affect our health has been recognized since biblical times. However, only relatively recently has humor become a subject of research. Prior to the 1960s the study of humor in the scientific community was considered non-professional. It was viewed as a subject not worthy of the serious researcher. As society becomes more aware of the benefits of humor, humor has become accepted as an effective intervention for healthcare providers and as an important area for investigation. Humor in nursing and health care in general, has gone from being covert to overt. Laughter Clubs and hospital humor programs are examples of successful humor interventions.

EXAM QUESTIONS

CHAPTER 2
Questions 10-18

Note: Choose the one option that BEST answers each question.

10. In the 19th century, scientist Herbert Spencer noted that laughter helped to

    a. eliminate pain.

    b. relieve tension.

    c. stimulate the immune system.

    d. overcome infection.

11. The first written reference to the importance of happiness and health occurs in the

    a. Bible.

    b. writings of Henri de Mondeville.

    c. writings of Laurent Joubert.

    d. *Saturday Evening Post.*

12. Dr. William Fry's interest in humor developed from his interest in

    a. pain management.

    b. psychology.

    c. verbal communication.

    d. nonverbal communication.

13. While dealing with the pain of ankylosing spondylitis, Norman Cousins found that 10 minutes of hearty laughter left him pain free for

    a. 2 hours.

    b. 2.5 hours.

    c. 3 hours.

    d. 3.5 hours.

14. Recent studies show that communication between the mind and body occurs through

    a. conscious thought and concentration.

    b. hormones, cytokines, and neuropeptides.

    c. the gastroenterology system.

    d. the parasympathetic nervous system.

15. Stereotypical depictions of nurses include the nurse as a servant or handmaiden, a nurturer, a sex-object, and

    a. a bearer of pain.

    b. an old battle-axe.

    c. an autonomous health provider.

    d. a scatterbrain.

16. The first nursing cartoons appeared in *RN* magazine in the

    a. early 1900s.

    b. 1920s.

    c. 1930s.

    d. 1940s.

17. The first nurse to publish a text on humor and the health professions was

    a. Karyn Buxman.

    b. Doug Fletcher.

    c. Alison Crane.

    d. Vera Robinson.

18. A relatively recent global influence in promoting the practical application of humor for health and world peace is

    a. the development of the American Association for Therapeutic Humor (AATH).

    b. the development of the World Laughter Tour (WLT).

    c. research findings by Dr. William Fry.

    d. Norman Cousins' book *Anatomy of an Illness as Perceived by the Patient.*

CHAPTER 3

DEVELOPMENT OF HUMOR APPRECIATION

CHAPTER OBJECTIVE

After completing this chapter, the reader will be able to describe how humor develops from infancy to adulthood.

LEARNING OBJECTIVES

After studying this chapter, the reader will be able to

1. identify how growth and development affects humor appreciation.

2. describe what children consider funny at different ages.

3. identify how changes in adulthood influence humor appreciation.

4. identify factors that influence the development of a sense of humor.

INTRODUCTION

Children and adults appreciate humor differently. Humor does not just happen; it is a product of development. Children do not laugh at things that they do not have the capacity to understand. The ability to appreciate humor and to utilize humor depends on experiences, cognitive development, language usage, ability to problem solve, and the ability to be creative. Much humor comes from incongruity. Because children do not have the experience that develops throughout life, they do not have the capacity to see incongruity with the same perspective as adults. This generally makes a child's sense of humor more limited than an adult's. One reason to explore how humor appreciation and use changes throughout development is that it offers us clues about general emotional and social well-being. As children age, the ability to appreciate and understand humor changes. This chapter will present general developmental information and then specific age-related behaviors. The age-groups covered range from infancy to old age.

GENERAL DEVELOPMENTAL INFORMATION

The job of childhood is learning. One way children learn is through play. Another way they learn is through humor. Humor helps increase vocabulary and pre-reading and reading skills. It helps strengthen a child's knowledge of the world, helps support creative thinking, builds social interaction skills, positively affects relationships between children, and helps build self-esteem.

Humor development follows maturational development. As children's knowledge goes from concrete to more abstract thinking, the type of humor children understand and participate in changes. If you pay attention to children's comprehension and reaction to humor, it can be seen that children find things funniest for the first few months after reaching new understanding, up to the first one or two years, after which that the particular form of humor seems less funny. As an example, riddles are often seen as funniest during first and second grade, and become less funny over time because they are too easily understood. With developmental learning, the riddle they used to think was funny becomes "dumb" or "stupid." Another way of stating this phenomenon is increased ease of understanding leads to decreased funniness.

Differences in gender, temperament and intelligence are noted in understanding, telling, and enjoying humor. A literature review by Peterson (2007) revealed that children between grades three and six who were considered funny by their peers and teachers had a superior range of intelligence. Children with higher verbal intelligence were more likely to comprehend jokes and cartoons. Those children with higher skillful and expressive use of language demonstrated high levels of humor responsiveness.

Gender difference has been noted in humor development and usage. Men seem to use humor more than women and men's humor tends to be more aggressive in nature. Women have reported using humor more as a coping mechanism than men (Peterson, 2007). Boys, especially sixth grade boys, were more likely to be considered funny by their peers and teachers than girls were.

THE EARLY YEARS: INFANCY TO AGE 2

It has been said that children laugh 400 times a day. Although there is no scientific research to back up that statistic, researchers do know that children appear to laugh far more than adults do. Humor development begins at a very early age. The beginning evidence of a sense of humor can be seen as early as the third or fourth month of age (Prerost, n.d.). Mimicking parents is an important function in

humor development because that is how children learn (Prerost, n.d). At this age, the expression of humor may come in the form of a smile or laughter. A smile is usually an indication of pleasure. It is also a means of communication. Ziv (1984) describes the smile as the "first form of positive communication" (p. 27). In infancy, a smile communicates the message "I feel good" (Ziv, 1984). Babies typically smile by age 3 months. People used to believe that infant smiles were a response to gas; however, they are now believed to be a response to fluctuations in a baby's level of arousal (Clark, 2002). By 6-weeks-old, most babies grin in response to a grinning face. A laughter response can be seen in children as young as age 3 months. One can see this response when a baby is tickled, kissed on the abdomen, or bounced (Clark, 2002).

Ziv (1984) states that until 8 weeks of age, the social smile occurs with recognition of human faces and voices in general. He further states that after 8 weeks of age, a baby's smile appears to be more selective, expressing recognition of a mother or father. An infant's smile appears to play an important part in the dialogue between parent and baby. The selective smile occurs at the time an infant moves from passivity to directed activity in other areas of life (Holland, 1982). By age 3 months, infants begin to respond to humorous events through nonreflexive laughter (Reddy, Williams, & Vaughan, 2002). In other words, an infant may respond with laughter or a smile to such phrases as "I'm going to get you," as well as to the physical stimulation of tickling or bouncing. The physical stimulation response results in laughter because it gives the immature nervous system a mild and pleasant jolt (Clark, 2002).

An interesting experiment by Holland (1982) noted that infants younger than the age of 8 months need to see the combination of forehead, nose, and two eyes to respond with a smile. A child will smile at a nodding Halloween mask that contains the proper features; however, he or she will not smile at the profile of a human face. As the infant ages, smiling only if the combination of forehead, nose, and eyes are visible will begin to change and the child will smile a smile that conveys recognition for loved adults. Whereas the child will smile at adults he or she recognizes, the response to strangers may result in expressions of anxiety.

One of the prerequisites for a sense of humor is the ability to recognize incongruences. A baby typically starts to demonstrate this ability between ages 6 and 9 months (Clark, 2002). Babies may respond to such behaviors as oinking like a pig or making "horse lips." Around age 7 months, babies begin to understand that objects are still there even if they cannot be seen; therefore, peekaboo and pop-up toys become funny. Playing "I'm going to get you" or kissing the baby's abdomen becomes even funnier because the baby is now able to anticipate what is coming.

An infant responds to a new stimulus with curiosity and attempts to manipulate the stimulus by touching or otherwise coming in contact with it. This behavior reflects an effort to understand and master the environment. An infant seems to respond with a smile to a new stimulus that has similarities with something the child finds familiar (Ziv, 1984), especially once they are sure that the stimulus is not harmful. If the stimulus is then presented on a continuous basis, the infant appears to become tired or bored with the effort to elicit a smile, and the smile disappears. This response may be a way of expressing the enjoyment of discovery and a sense of victory in problem solving.

As children continue to develop, they begin to recognize and understand events that are incongruent. By age 11 or 12 months, infants laugh at funny faces and sounds or funny events, such as a person waddling like a duck or an adult sucking from a baby bottle (Reddy, Williams, & Vaughan, 2002). By age 10 months, many children have started to initiate humor and begin laughing even before the end of a humorous event.

Humor development can be understood by looking at Piaget's developmental tasks. The first task is sensorimotor, which occurs from birth to age 2 years. During this stage, the child begins to understand that objects continue to exist even when they cannot be touched, seen, or heard. They also begin to understand that things do not just happen. They are caused by something or someone. Children recognize humor when they have developed "representational capabilities sufficiently to allow them to represent things as other than they appear" (Cundall, 2007, p. 210). As children age, they begin to realize that they can affect events by behaving in certain ways. Reddy et al. (2002) note that children begin to recognize that they can cause others to laugh by clowning and teasing. Piaget mentions that one of his daughters at 1½ years of age pretended to eat with no food in front of her. His second daughter, at about the same age, pretended to brush her teeth with her finger as if it were a toothbrush. These behaviors were accompanied by a smile and laughter (Newman & Newman, 1999).

AGES 2 TO 7

Piaget's preoperational thought developmental stage occurs approximately between ages 2 and 7. During this stage, a child has increased language skills and can differentiate thought from action (Howe, 1993). Children who have reached the preoperational stage and have an image-based representational capacity have the ability to find humor in acting on one object as if it were another object (Martin, 1989) – for example, a child who laughs at a picture of a hippopotamus trying to get on a pair of pants. After all, hippopotamuses don't wear pants, people do. Another example is the following joke: "Why did the elephant paint her toenails red?" "So she could hide in the strawberry patch."

One function of humor is to release tension (Klein, 1992). At age 2, children begin to experi-

Note. From BeingFive.blogspot.com. Used with permission.

ence many conflict situations. They start learning that their views and goals are often not shared by the adults in their lives. The use of humorous situations presented in books or cartoons appears to help them learn that difficult problems can be resolved in constructive ways.

Two-year-olds typically like stories based on experiences that they find physically challenging, such as walking, running, dressing, undressing, and bathing themselves (Klein, 1992). Being able to laugh at the silly mistakes depicted in storybooks helps children realize that they can or have developed mastery over some of these behaviors. Humor helps children explore and cope with issues that can be a source of anxiety, which is one reason why most preschool and kindergarten children laugh at potty humor (Barasch, 1999). Humor helps learning because it motivates, arouses, and stimulates the child's cognitive processes (Klein, 1992; McGhee, 1989). Flatter (1995) states that 2- and 3-year-olds are prone to copycat humor, which is part of a pattern of modeling behaviors.

During the preschool years, children attempt to master spoken language. This attempt can make nonsense words a source of enjoyment (Barasch, 1999). Children learning to use language sometimes deliberately use a wrong word as they play with their own and others' reactions to language. After all, one way to learn a new skill is to play

with it. Children may distort words, make up words, or cause nonsense words to rhyme and demonstrate joy in their ability to make something seem funny. Although they have not yet figured out what makes a joke funny, they begin to tell jokes and riddles.

One word of caution when working with preschoolers: there may be a very fine line between what is funny and what is frightening to them (Flatter, 1995). A clown wearing exaggerated face paint and a bright orange wig might elicit reactions of fear rather than amusement. Activities that are too out of the ordinary or playacting that goes on too long may cause feelings of anxiety.

Kindergarten children find almost everything funny (Howe, 1993). This age-group is especially fond of clowns, funny stories about animals and people, and bathroom humor. Bathroom humor can be as simple as mentioning the word "underwear." Kindergartners' humor seems to reflect their silliness and lack of "cognitive sophistication" (Howe, 1993).

To investigate the ability of young children to understand and appreciate cognitively oriented humor, Klein (n.d.) studied the relationship between humor comprehension and three forms of humor appreciation. The results of this study indicate that children between 5 and 6 years old are able to describe or explain joking relationships, demonstrating comprehension of intended humor.

Bariaud (1989) notes that children between ages 3 and 5 find humor in things that represent incongruity in appearances, such as a cow taking a bath and washing himself with a scrub brush. At approximately age 6, a change in joking style takes place. Prior to age 6, children seem to enjoy their own inventions of humor, and the humor tends to be spontaneous, original, and relatively crude (Bariaud, 1989). At age 6 children begin to show an interest in ready-made jokes. This interest continues to develop between ages 7 and 10 (Bariaud, 1989).

By around the age of 6 they begin to find the stringing of silly words (ludicrous juxtapositions), play on words, or logical flaws funny. Also around the age of 6 or 7 children begin to understand that some words can have two meanings. This understanding of double meaning, like sale or sail, leads to better understanding of riddles that they may have been telling for the last year or so. Examples of the type of riddles these children might tell over and over are:

What cake can you drink coffee from? A cup cake.

What boats can you always buy at a reduced price? Sale (sail) boats.

A banana and an apple got married, but they argued all the time. So the banana split.

Peterson (2008) studied humor styles and how humor might be used by first-graders as a buffer against rejection and depression. She examined aggressive humor and self-enhancing humor and the personal effects of these humor styles on the students and how others perceived them. Her study revealed that boys were more likely to use humor than girls at this age. Boys are more likely to use aggressive humor but this behavior is often not seen as aggressive by their teachers. Young girls who engage in aggressive humor, however, are seen as having more aggressive behavior than their peers. It is hypothesized that this trend might be due to the expectation that girls do not use aggressive humor.

Peer-reported aggressive humor seems to correlate with teacher-reported aggressive behavior. In other words, kids who use aggressive humor are perceived as being more aggressive and having more social problems than kids who do not use this style of humor. Aggressive humor might be a clue to check for potential social problems and peer rejection. The study by Peterson did not reveal a high use of self-enhancing humor. This finding might be because self-enhancing humor is a higher cognitive skill.

At age 7, a change in humor appreciation occurs (Bariaud, 1989). Seven-year-olds may respond in a serious manner to riddles that 1 year earlier would have caused laughter (Bariaud, 1989). Watching 7-year-olds try to decipher a cartoon so that the incongruity in it made sense led Bariaud (1989) to conclude that children of this age have not mastered the "convention according to which such cartoons purposefully distort things in order to be funny" (p. 38). In this study using cartoons, Bariaud (1989) found that 7-year-olds would explain that the cartoon could not be funny because "it can't be like that" (p. 38). Not all 7-year-olds responded in this manner, but a significant number did. Howe (1993) notes that this age-group finds cartoons, clowns, and riddles enjoyable. They tend to like patterns of riddles, like elephant or knock-knock jokes, and may tell them for weeks. They delight in trying to outwit adults with the riddles (Barasch, 1999; Howe, 1993).

Joking is a way of connecting with others. Adults use humor in social situations to improve relationships. Children around 6 and 7 years old begin to realize that humor can help them gain acceptance, approval or, if nothing else, someone's attention (Barasch, 1999).

Adults are not the only ones who use humor to cope with fears and anxieties. Children also find that humor helps them cope with these emotions. As children start exploring the outside world, humor works to defuse some of the anxiety they experience (Barasch, 1999). Jokes that make fun of others, such as those with disabilities, may be a way for children to deal with their own fears of being injured, disabled, or somehow different from others. Laughter may be a way of soothing anxiety, but it might not be connected with humor. As an example, a child may laugh when another child trips or something angers the teacher. This laughter might be a way of distancing themselves from the fears aroused by an uncomfortable situation.

AGES 7 TO 12

According to Piaget, children ages 7 to 12 are in the concrete operational stage. Howe (1993) notes that third-grade children begin to demonstrate less fear of authority, and this seems to lead to teachers becoming a source of humor. A study by Socha (1994) investigated the use of prosocial and antisocial humor. Antisocial humor refers to the type of humor that pokes fun at different people. It can be hurtful to an individual or a group. He discovered that children up to fourth grade tended to use more prosocial humor than antisocial humor. If antisocial behavior was used, it was usually used by boys and aimed at other children. Up until eighth grade, children were more likely to use humor that had some decorum when communicating with teachers. The eighth-grade children who demonstrated less polite humor, such as teasing the teacher about hair loss, seemed to be comfortable with the teacher they were teasing.

Socha (1994) found a significant change from prosocial to antisocial joke telling in the fourth grade. This change was significantly greater for boys than for girls. The boys' behavior showed an increased tendency to make fun of others. Girls also tended to make fun of others, but not to the same extent as did the boys.

Howe (1993) states that fourth graders tend to use humor that revolves around their peers, with increased emphasis on the opposite sex and friends' mistakes. They do not see other students

getting in trouble as funny, as is the tendency of those in third grade. A study by Shade (1991) found that fourth-grade children enjoyed jokes and riddles over puns and satire. This is probably indicative of their cognitive level, which is not developed enough to enjoy puns and satire. Children of this age still take comments very literally (Howe, 1993; Shade, 1991).

By fifth grade, children begin to show a decrease in slapstick humor and an increase in more social humor. According to Howe (1993), the humor found in others making mistakes greatly increases among this age-group. This behavior was noticed in fourth graders by Socha (1994).

By fourth or fifth grade, there is a noticeable difference between boys' humor and girls' humor. Around age 10, boys tend to tell jokes that are sexual or physically violent, such as 'How do you make a cat sound like a dog? You pour gasoline on it and light it with a match and it goes, "WHOOOF!"' (*A Prairie Home Companion Pretty Good Joke Book,* 2005, p. 156) Girls at the same age like humor that is more verbally aggressive rather than physically violent. They tend to tease each other about boyfriends and "act like caricatures of the vamps they see on television soap operas." Despite the differences, jokes are an indirect way for each group to deal with the issues they are most concerned about, such as their sexuality (Kutner, n.d.).

An interesting study by Graves (2008) describes story-telling abilities of children. This study revealed the use of humor in 8- and 9-year-olds during the story-telling experience. Interestingly, this is the only age-group that used playful humor in the process of writing their stories. Students who were younger and those who were older did not employ humor to tell their stories. It is believed that humor helped the child tell the story in a way that separated him from the events being shared, especially in areas like curiosity in parental sexual activity or behaviors seen as not socially acceptable. The author asserts that the use of humor in this age-group demonstrates an ability to recognize discrepancies and employ them effectively for comic effect.

Sixth-grade humor shows a continued increase in the use of social humor. Howe (1993) notes that mistakes made by others, especially peers, tops the list of things that are funny. Cognitive understanding improves in this age-group and incongruities are better understood. Crude behavior and grossness are likely to be seen as humorous, especially by boys. Boys also tend to find body noises funny, just as they did in first grade (Howe, 1993).

PREADOLESCENCE AND ADOLESCENCE

Around the age of 12, children move into Piaget's fourth stage: formal operational thought. By this age, children can think hypothetically. Although it is a gradual development, the ability to think abstractly becomes more fully developed, allowing the child to think of a number of scenarios when asked how things might be different. At this age, children begin to actively use humor for coping with stressful life events (Fuhr, 2002). They also begin to make jokes about their situation. For example, a 12-year-old deliberately uses humor to deal with an upcoming heart transplant (Dowling, 2002).

Fuhr (2002) studied the form and function of humor in children ages 12 to 16 from Copenhagen. He studied students in two different schools to see if there was a difference between humor use and appreciation in students from the country versus students from a town. Fuhr's study indicated that some types of jokes were preferred more by one group than another. The differences appeared to be connected with life situations. This study confirms Kutner's (n.d.) comment that children's humor seems to be connected to the developmental tasks with which they are struggling. The three areas that had notable differences were:

- "plans for the future," which was of higher interest to town children;

- "boyfriends or girlfriends," which was also of higher interest in children from town; and

- "other," which was of higher interest to children from the country

(Fuhr, 2002).

Sex-related jokes were found to have a high level of interest for 12- to 13-year-olds in Fuhr's 2002 study. Sex was the most important theme for 12-year-olds in particular. Sex was more important for boys than for girls. As noted earlier, responses to humor follows growth and development levels. Boys at the age of 12 are usually more interested in sexual things than girls, so it follows that they would find sexual jokes funnier than girls would.

With increased age, the use of coping humor increases (Fuhr, 2002). This is believed to be due to increased experiences and the witnessing of others using humor to cope.

Very few studies explore the development of the type of humor enjoyed in adolescence. What we do know is that, as children develop, gain experience, and synthesize information, their appreciation and understanding of humor changes and becomes more adult-like. Klause (1987) notes that teens appear to enjoy puns. This enjoyment of puns decreases as individuals move into adulthood. However, the cognitive process of formulating the pun seems to bring enjoyment to the one who designs it (Klause, 1987).

ADULTHOOD

As with other areas of human development, when a person reaches adulthood, humor development seems to stop. However, humor responses and usage continue to develop and change as a person continues to age. It is fair to assume that, with changes in cognitive abilities, social relationships, psychological concerns and needs, attitudes, and coping with issues such as life events, humor appreciation will change over time. However, the research on how humor appreciation of adults changes over time is limited (Ruch, McGhee, & Hehl, 1990), although a few studies have explored how older adults respond to humor in different situations. Listed below are descriptions of two examples of humor that are commonly seen in adults.

McGhee, Ruch, and Hehl (cited in Ruch et al., 1990) suggest a model of humor development in adulthood. According to this model, there is a strong link between age, differences in personality variables such as intolerance of ambiguity and sensation seeking, and appreciation of humorous materials such as cartoons and jokes. Ruch et al. (1990) report that studies demonstrate that more-conservative people find "incongruity-resolution humor funnier and less aversive than do more liberal individuals" (p. 348). The opposite is true of nonsense humor. Individuals who have an increased intolerance to ambiguity appreciate incongruity-resolution humor more than nonsense humor. This finding is consistent with the view that these personality dimensions are most likely to dislike or avoid novel, complex, incongruous, or ambiguous events that leave a person in a state of high subjective uncertainty.

The following is an example of the differences between the two types of humor.

Incongruity-resolution: A traffic cop pulled alongside a speeding car on the motorway. Glancing into the car, he was astounded to see that the young lady, who was driving, was knitting.

Realizing that she was oblivious to his flashing lights and siren, the policeman wound down his window, turned on his loudspeaker and yelled, "PULL OVER!"

"NO," the young lady yelled back, "IT'S A SCARF!"

Nonsense Humor: Two elephants are sitting in a bathtub. One elephant says to the other, "Pass the soap." The other elephant responds, "No soap. Radio."

Cross-sectional studies demonstrate age differences in the personality dimensions of conservatism, sensation seeking, and intolerance of ambiguity (Ruch et al., 1990). Much of the data indicates that sensation seeking peaks in the late teens or early 20s and then decreases with age. Conservatism commonly begins to appear in the late 20s and increases until past age 60.

Ruch et al. conducted a cross-sectional study of 4,292 subjects to test the McGhee, Ruch, and Hehl model. The study included 3,057 males ages 14 to 66 and 1,235 females ages 14 to 54. The researchers recognized that cohort differences might exist among the subjects, in that the older adults might always have been more conservative and less sensation seeking than the younger adults. The researchers were looking to discover if appreciation of incongruity-resolution humor increased with age, beginning in the late 20s or early 30s, and if appreciation of nonsense humor changed with a progressive drop after age 30.

The researchers found that their results were relatively consistent with the McGhee, Ruch, and Hehl model. They also found a few areas of interest. First, 14- to 16-year-olds demonstrated relatively high incongruity-resolution scores. Then, nonsense humor scales increased until the late 20s, when the incongruity-resolution scores began to gradually increase. Those individuals in their 40s showed a sharp increase in incongruity-resolution humor appreciation. This was consistent with the increase in conservatism.

All ages younger than the 29 to 31 age-group, (except the 14- to 16-year-olds, who found incongruity-resolution humor funnier than nonsense humor), judged the two humor structures comparably funny (Ruch et al., 1990). This pattern began to change with an increase in incongruity-resolution humor appreciation. One drawback of this study is that it was cross-sectional and not longitudinal, so the changes found might reflect age-group differences rather than changes that occur as people age. A longitudinal study following the same group of adults over time would be more likely to answer the question of how humor might change as people age.

A study from Baycrest Centre for Geriatric Care (2003) in Toronto found that humor appreciation does not change with age. However, this study found that comprehension of complex forms of humor does diminish with age. The study was conducted using 20 healthy older adults, whose average age was 73, and 17 healthy younger adults, whose average age was 28. To understand the results, it is helpful to understand the tasks requested of the participants.

The participants were asked to complete three separate humor tests: differentiating humorous statements from neutral statements, joke and story completion, and nonverbal cartoon appreciation. The first test looked at humor appreciation. It consisted of 21 humorous and 7 neutral statements. Examples of humorous statements included a sign in a tailor shop that read, "Please have a fit upstairs," and a sign in a hotel that read, "Guests are invited to take advantage of the chambermaid" (Baycrest Centre for Geriatric Care, 2003, p. 10). One of the neutral statements was a sign in a hotel that read, "Visitors are requested to turn off the lights when they leave the room."

The second test consisted of having the participants choose the correct punch lines for 16 incomplete joke stems. Only one of the four endings offered was the correct humorous punch line. The third test consisted of 10 different cartoon drawings. Each cartoon had a series of four similar drawings, but only one had a funny detail. Participants were asked to choose the funny version.

This study found that older adults did just as well as the younger participants on the first test. However, the older adults made significant mistakes on the two more cognitively challenging tests. The difficulty in comprehending more complex forms of humor may be related to age-related changes in the frontal lobes. Biological evidence suggests that frontal lobe functions may be the first to decline with age (Baycrest Centre for Geriatric Care, 2003). Despite their difficulty comprehending more complex humor, the older participants reacted appropriately with a smile or laugh when they did understand the humor. This suggests that the humor processing related to other regions in the brain remains intact.

The researchers of this study caution that the study was just preliminary. Overinterpretation of the results needs to be avoided. Limitations of the study include small sample size and a lack of investigation of cohort differences in the type of humor preferred, social setting, or health – all of which contribute to our response to humorous situations.

Two studies reported in Martin's (2007) text looked at older adults' responses compared to younger adults. In one study using the Multidimensional Sense of Humor Scale, older participants reported producing and appreciating humor somewhat more than the younger adults. The older adults were also more likely to use humor to cope with stress. They were also more likely to have a negative reaction toward humorous people.

Another study indicated that older adults had significantly lower scores on both affiliative and aggressive humor than younger adults (Martin, 2007). This finding indicates that older adults are less likely to engage in friendly joking (affiliative) as well as aggressive humor than younger adults. The indication is that older adults may be less likely to engage in friendly banter or laughter and also less likely to use humor that is disparaging, ridiculing, or manipulative. The study also found that older women (not men) used self-enhancing humor more than younger adults, indicating a more humorous outlook on life and greater use of perspective-taking as well as coping humor.

McMahan (2008) discovered that children reacted differently to clowning than older adults during a trip with a group called Clowns without Borders. McMahan studied theatrical clowning and became interested in joining Clowns without Borders on one of their trips to South Africa. The group found that children's laughter was explosive and high energy. In contrast, the elderly patients they visited were slow to laugh, less explosive, but had a depth that the children's laughter never seemed to reach. The laughter connected the performer to the participant. They were also willing participants in creating humor, which generated laughter from the audience in the nursing homes visited.

Table 3-1 summarizes the developmental stages of humor by age, as noted by the above studies.

SENSE OF HUMOR

The previous section discussed the development of humor appreciation, but did not really address the issue of developing a sense of humor. If humor is an abstract concept, a sense of humor is even more abstract. A sense of humor can be considered a personality trait. Some people are considered to have a good sense of humor, others are thought to be humorless. However, how we define someone else's sense of humor might depend on the correlation between what we find funny and what the other person finds funny. If we think something is funny and the other person agrees, we perceive they have a good sense of humor. If, on the other hand, what we find funny the other person does not see as funny, we perceive they have no or a "bad" sense of humor. Martin (2007) notes that saying someone has a sense of humor implies that "we have frequently observed this person engaging in a variety of humor-related behaviors" during a number of different situations (p. 219). The concept of a sense of humor might be viewed "as a socially constructed description of a person's typical humor-related conduct" (Martin, 2007, p. 219).

We will leave the idea of measuring sense of humor to personality psychologists and review those aspects about which there is more concrete knowledge, such as those factors that might influence a person's sense of humor. From the studies that have been conducted, it appears that a sense of humor contains genetic and environmental influences (Martin, 2007). The types of things people laugh at seem to be influenced by experiences within and outside of their family of origin. On the other hand, genetic factors seem most prevalent when looking at characteristics such as the tendency to laugh and smile frequently and other behaviors denoting positive emotionality.

Martin (2007) discusses a number of studies looking at environment versus genetic contributions. It is apparent that one of the influential environmental aspects of sense of humor development is the family. Children appear to learn to express and enjoy humor during their early relationships with their parents and other family members. Parents who like to joke and laugh a lot are a model for children and are more likely to reinforce their children's attempts to use humor. The belief that parents and family influence sense of humor is referred to as the Modeling/Reinforcement Hypothesis. The other hypothesis that might explain how some children develop a sense of humor is called the Stress and Coping Hypothesis. This premise suggests that children may develop a sense of humor as a way of coping with distress. For children dealing with a difficult family environment, humor might be a way of releasing angry feelings or gaining attention and approval from parents who may usually be rejecting and non-nurturing. Martin notes that there is evidence to support both hypotheses.

The discussion of personality and behavioral correlates of children's sense of humor is long and involved. The end results of the studies that have been conducted depended on how sense of humor is defined. It also depended on the age of the child. As noted above, aggressive humor is more likely seen in certain age-groups, particularly fourth graders, and mostly the male students. One study

TABLE 3-1: DEVELOPMENTAL STAGES OF BEHAVIOR BY AGE (1 OF 2)

Cognitive Stage and Age	Developmental Behaviors
Sensorimotor	
6 weeks	• Baby grins at a grinning face. • Baby smiles in recognition of human faces and voices.
8 weeks	• Baby becomes more selective, grinning only at mother or father. • Baby attempts a type of dialogue with parents.
3 months	• Baby begins to smile or laugh at certain phrases, tickling, or bouncing.
6 to 9 months	• Baby begins to recognize incongruences. • Baby may smile or laugh at pig sounds or funny faces.
Around 7 months	• Peekaboo and pop-up toys become funny. • Baby begins to anticipate reactions, so playing "I'm going to get you" or kissing the abdomen becomes funnier.
8 months and younger	• The combination of forehead, nose, and eyes are needed for smile response.
8 months and older	• Combination of facial feature response decreases, and the child smiles at recognition of loved adults.
10 months	• Child may initiate humor.
11 or 12 months	• Child laughs at funny faces, sounds, or a person making animal movements such as waddling like a duck.
Preoperational	
2 to 5 years	• Child is prone to copycat humor (ages 2 to 3). • Increased language skills and recognition of differences between thought and action can lead to the ability to find humor in pictures or stories of incongruent behavior. • Child laughs at silly mistakes depicted in books. • Child begins to understand that humor can be used to help cope with new and difficult situations. • Child likes to experiment with new words and sounds and uses nonsense words to make humor. • Child demonstrates joy in making things seem funny. • Child begins to tell jokes and riddles. • Things that are outrageous, such as clowns with exaggerated face paint and bright orange wigs, might cause fear rather than amusement.
5 to 6 years	• Child finds almost everything funny. • Child laughs at insults, practical jokes, and accidents that happen to others. • Child is fond of clowns and funny stories. • Child likes bathroom humor. • Child is able to explain joking relationships. • Child begins to show an interest in ready-made jokes.

TABLE 3-1: DEVELOPMENTAL STAGES OF BEHAVIOR BY AGE (2 OF 2)	
Concrete Operational	
7 years	• Child seems to become more serious.
	• Humor is more reality based.
	• Child likes cartoons, riddles, and clowns.
	• Child likes to try to outwit adults with riddles.
7 to 12 years	• Child begins to demonstrate less fear of authority, making teachers a source of humor.
	• Child tends to use mainly prosocial humor (between ages 7 and 9).
	• Child laughs at reality-oriented, more-complex riddles that fit into the child's understanding of the world.
	• Child exhibits an increase in antisocial humor and an increase in making fun of others (9-year-olds).
	• Child enjoys jokes and riddles over puns and satire.
	• Child begins to move from slapstick humor to more social humor (10-year-olds).
	• Boys' humor differs from girls' humor (9- and 10-year-olds).
	• Child demonstrates increased use of social humor (11- and 12-year-olds).
	• Child still sees mistakes by others as funny.
	• Boys tend to find body noises funny, similar to first grade enjoyment.
Formal Operational	
12 years	• Gradual ability to think abstractly leads to increased use of humor as a coping mechanism.
	• Child exhibits increased enjoyment of sexual jokes, especially with boys.
Adolescence	• Use of coping humor increases.
	• Adolescent still enjoys puns.
	• Adolescent has a high incongruity-resolution score (14- to 16-year-olds).
Adulthood	• Conservative individuals appreciate incongruity-resolution humor.
	• Enjoyment of nonsense humor increases with age.
Older Adulthood	• Humor appreciation does not change with age.
	• Understanding of complex humor decreases.

Note. Data for this table was accumulated from Barasch, 1999; Bariaud, 1989; Clark, 2002; Herzog, 2004; McGhee, 1989; Reddy, Williams & Vaughan, 2002; Ruch, McGhee, & Hehl, 1990; Socha, 1994; and Ziv, 1984.

discussed by Martin revealed that 4- and 5-year-old children with more advanced language skills were more likely to initiate humor when interacting with their peers. Studies with older children revealed that the "high-humor" children might be more likely to be labeled attention seekers by adults and may be seen as disruptive and unruly; however they tended to be very popular with their class-mates. As children age, the initiation of humor is more likely to happen as ways of being accepted by peers. The things children find funny develops and changes as their sense of humor develops and changes. When it comes to measuring behaviors that can be labeled "sense of humor" it seems to depend on how sense of humor is defined.

CASE STUDY

*K*athy is a 10-year-old girl admitted to the unit with osteomyelitis. She has a bulky dressing with continuous antibiotic irrigation and IV antibiotics. She is on bed rest with bathroom privileges with no weight-bearing on the affected leg. She is fearful and cries during her dressing changes. The social worker and nurses are concerned about how to help Kathy deal with her admission and disease process. They decided to try adding humor to her treatment plan.

Questions

1. What assessments would you make to find out how Kathy uses humor?

2. Give specific examples of the type of humor appropriate for her age-group.

Discussion

The best way to assess someone's use of humor is to ask. The best time to ask is when the child is calm – definitely not during the dressing change or right before or after the dressing change. Assessment can include the following:

- What do you find funny?
- Tell me one of your favorite jokes.
- What TV shows do you find fun to watch?
- Think back to the last time you laughed. Share with me what it was that made you laugh.
- What movies make you laugh?

If the staff is attempting to use humor as a method of decreasing her distress during the dressing change, then finding a movie that she finds funny, or one with similar humor, is helpful. At the age of 10 she will most likely enjoy movies that have scenes in it that pertain to relationships. Many 10-year-olds enjoy sitcoms and humorous family shows. Stories that have verbally aggressive humor might be something she will enjoy. Whereas boys around 10 years of age like jokes that are sexually or physically violent, girls usually do not, so that is important to keep in mind when choosing funny material for Kathy. One set of books that has been recommended for children around 10 is the Melanie Martin series written by Carol Weston. The books are humorous, and Melanie travels with her family, so the reader also learns about different areas of the country and the world. Other recommended books include Henry Reed books by Keith Robertson. The internet is a valuable means for identifying appropriate material.

SUMMARY

The development of humor from childhood to adulthood has received attention from the scientific community. One of the first people to research the development of humor in children was Paul McGhee. Since then, others have researched development of humor from different perspectives, such as Fuhr's research into the use of coping humor in children ages 12 to 16. The understanding of humorous material changes as children develop cognitively. This development of humor continues into adulthood, as the events that trigger a humor response take on different meanings. Research suggests that older adults do not lose their ability to appreciate humor, but changes in the frontal lobe can lead to diminished ability to understand complex humor. Studies also suggest that humor serves different functions for adults at different periods of the lifespan. It seems that younger adults have more of a need to use humor to express aggression in socially acceptable ways, establish relationships, and test one's social standing in their peer group. On the other hand, older adults, especially women, are more likely to employ humor to cope with stress and maintain a positive outlook on life.

By understanding humor development, mental health providers can use humor comprehension to help determine developmental progress. As noted in

Petersons' study, it might also help in indicating problems with aggressive behavior. It can also serve as a guideline for developing educational programs.

"I was performing a complete physical, including the visual acuity test. I placed the patient twenty feet from the chart and began, "Cover your right eye with your hand." He read the 20/20 line perfectly. "Now your left." Again, a flawless read. "Now both," I requested. There was silence. He couldn't even read the large E on the top line. I turned and discovered that he had done exactly what I had asked: he was standing there with both his eyes covered. I was laughing too hard to finish the exam.

– Dr. Matthew Theodropolous Villanus, Worcester, MA

EXAM QUESTIONS

CHAPTER 3
Questions 19-27

Note: Choose the one option that BEST answers each question.

19. It is most correct to say that humor development occurs

    a. in a linear manner.

    b. through maturational development.

    c. faster in boys than in girls.

    d. according to genetic factors.

20. According to Holland's experiment, infants younger than age 8 months smile in response to

    a. the profile of a human face.

    b. a mask of a one-eyed monster.

    c. recognition of incongruence.

    d. a view of a forehead, two eyes, and a nose.

21. Two year old children who have reached the preoperational stage now have the ability to find humor in

    a. silly mistakes depicted in books.

    b. bathroom humor.

    c. tickling people.

    d. making fun of others.

22. According to Flatter, the use of humorous situations in cartoons and storybooks allows 2- to 3-year-olds to

    a. learn and repeat ready-made jokes.

    b. use copycat humor to model behavior.

    c. change feelings by increasing anxiety.

    d. develop a sense of incongruence.

23. Because of their cognitive level, children around the age of 6 or 7 years old can now

    a. have fun experimenting with new words and sounds.

    b. enjoy nonsense humor.

    c. have a better understanding of riddles.

    d. laugh at silly mistakes depicted in books.

24. The use of sexual humor is more prominent with boys at the age of

    a. 2 years old.

    b. 4 years old.

    c. 8 years old.

    d. 12 years old.

25. Adolescent humor differs from humor for children younger than age 12. In adolescent humor

    a. incongruencies are not well understood.

    b. sex-related jokes and puns are less prevalent.

    c. the adolescent is more likely to use humor to cope.

    d. spontaneous and original jokes are common.

26. As adults increase in conservatism, their appreciation of humor becomes more

    a. sexually oriented.

    b. nonsense oriented.

    c. incongruity-resolution oriented

    d. bathroom-humor oriented.

27. Sense of humor development most likely occurs through the influence of

    a. genetic and environmental influences.

    b. genetic influences only.

    c. family influence only.

    d. environmental influences.

CHAPTER 4

INTRODUCTION TO USING HUMOR IN THE HEALTHCARE SETTING

CHAPTER OBJECTIVES

After completing this chapter, the reader will be able to explain how humor can be used in the healthcare setting to benefit patients and their providers.

LEARNING OBJECTIVES

After studying this chapter, the reader will be able to

1. describe the three roles of humor in health care as defined by Buxman.

2. discuss the importance of humor as a prevention for burnout.

3. describe how healthcare workers use humor to connect with their patients.

4. describe how humor can be incorporated into patient care.

5. articulate the purpose of taking a humor assessment.

6. recognize the differences between helpful and hurtful humor.

INTRODUCTION

Humor is an important component for helping to maintain health. This fact has been demonstrated in research as well as in the personal experiences of most individuals. The following chapters will share the details of how humor has been shown physiologically and psychosocially helpful. This chapter will give you background in the role humor plays in helping health care professionals connect with and care for individuals. Through the years, healthcare providers have been cautioned that humor may not be appropriate when someone is feeling ill or dealing with life-threatening situations. However, even individuals who are dying appreciate the use of humor (Herth, 1995). Not only is humor an important tool to use with patients, but it is also an important tool for providers to use to deal with the tensions and stress of their job. This chapter explores issues concerning the appropriate use of humor. It also discusses the way in which healthcare providers use and discuss humor with their patients and each other and as a method for decreasing the potential for burnout.

USING HUMOR TO SURVIVE BEING A HEALTHCARE PROVIDER

In this era of decreasing staff, decreasing healthcare reimbursement, and increasing workload, how would providers survive without humor? For example, consider the following scenario: The nurse has seven acutely ill patients, a doctor is screaming for assistance with a procedure, a patient is in pain and constantly on her call light, and down the hall a patient with dementia is yelling, "Help me, God. Oh please, help me, God." What do you do? Screaming is out, although that might be exactly what the nurse feels like doing. What would happen if the nurse took one moment, got on the intercom to the room of the patient with dementia, and said, "This is God. Now go to sleep." That happened one night at a small, rural hospital in southeast Arizona. The patient, who had barely slept since she arrived at the hospital, fell asleep and slept the rest of the evening.

Robinson (1991) notes that "the health professional's need for humor is as great as that of the client" (p. 73). Stressors arise daily in the healthcare setting. Staff must choose how they respond to those stressors. There are many ways to deal with the stress of work. Humor is just one of them; the other options may be unacceptable in a healthcare setting. For example, staff have no time for meditation or relaxation exercises, and yelling or crying is viewed as unprofessional. Humor can be helpful, even if the staff member just keeps the "joke" to herself or himself. However, shared humor helps diffuse the situation even more.

Buxman (1998) describes three main functions of humor in the healthcare settings. These functions are: psychological, social, and communication.

Psychological

Humor releases tension and gives the user a different perspective on his or her situation. The release of tension can increase creativity and leads to "perceptual flexibility" that can help increase a healthcare worker's sense of control.

Mirthfully exaggerating might help put the situation into perspective. For example: A patient pushes the call light to complain about the lousy food just as you are heading down the hallway to give a stat medication, hang blood, and check on a patient with symptoms of dyspnea. You ask yourself, "How could this be worse?" Perhaps it could be. The patient could be calling the local news station to report a food-poisoning outbreak at your hospital as well. That is a start, but now exaggerate again: "How could this be worse?" The news station might be a national affiliate willing to televise the late-breaking news flash on the national evening news. Yes, that would be worse, but exaggerate it one more time: "How could this be worse?" The patient might be the news anchor's brother-in-law, and the anchor is now bringing in the whole news crew to do a 1-hour exposé on the terrible food at your hospital! That would definitely be worse! The goal of this exercise is not to laugh hysterically every time something stressful comes up but to reframe the event and put it in its proper perspective and maybe even generate a slight smile.

This exercise works well as a mind-storming event when the nurse is dealing with the stressor alone, or as a brain-storming event when several people are dealing with the same challenge (Buxman, 2000b).

Note. From Nurstoon.com. Used with permission.

Social

The sharing of amusement creates a bond. It also helps to establish an equal relationship and decreases the sense of perceived hierarchy, even if for only a moment. It is difficult to remain angry or upset at someone with whom you have shared humor.

An operating room manager shared the following story regarding orientation of a new employee.

When a new nurse comes to our department we do the usual formal greeting, but when we finally get a chance to sit down together as a group, usually over a bite to eat, I ask each person to share their most embarrassing moment or horror story. It always gets lots of laughs, and someone can always out-do another's story. In the end, the group seems more cohesive. The new person is more of an insider as a result of having shared in these experiences. (Buxman, 2008, p. 72)

Communication

Humor allows a person to express concern, fear, or anger in a jestful manner, thus being able to "save face" if the recipient of the message does not respond kindly. The person making the comment can say, "I was only joking." If a patient makes this comment, the healthcare worker can look beyond the patient's words for an underlying emotion or meaning. If the patient is fearful or anxious, the nurse can devise an intervention to help the patient deal with the situation.

Effective use of humor can also help prevent the ever present possibility of burnout. Healthcare providers deal with the reality of illness, suffering, and death on a daily basis. Compassion and caring can leave a healthcare provider vulnerable to feelings of sympathy. Sympathy causes a person to feel another person's pain, and can leave a healthcare provider vulnerable to feelings of fear, anxiety, anger, or depression. Humor works as a tool to allow the care provider a more detached perspective. As Christina Maslach (1982, cited in Wooten,

1996) states, "Sometimes things are so frustrating that to keep from crying, you laugh at a situation that may not be funny. You laugh but in your heart you know what's really happening. Nevertheless, you do it because your own needs are important. We're all human beings and have to be ourselves" (p. 19).

Being able to project feelings that arise from frustration or sadness is to find a target. One area of frustration and anger for hospital workers is administration. They can become a safe target, as long as none are around at the time. The following joke was shared with Buxman (2008) by an operating room manager.

How many CEOs does it take to wallpaper a nurse's station? Two, if you slice them thin enough (p. 72).

One major factor in burnout is a sense of powerlessness. This sensation can leave a person feeling frustrated, angry, or hopeless. Some people give in to that feeling and leave the profession as a means of emotional protection. Others are more resilient and experience less burnout. Resilient individuals are able to withstand the strains of life's stressors and bounce back from adversity by using coping methods such as humor. Studies indicate that teachers who used humor to cope with stress of teaching had less feelings of depersonalization, exhaustion, and low personal accomplishment than those who did not use humor to cope (Tumkaya, 2007). However, those using aggressive humor and self-defeating humor were more likely to experience burnout.

A study looking at the factors relating to the level of burnout experienced by psychologists working for agencies versus independent practitioners discovered that both groups felt that maintaining a sense of humor was an important measure to prevent burnout (Rupert & Kent, 2007). The use of humor was seen as a cognitive strategy for keeping work demands in perspective.

One type of humor that commonly develops during times of high stress is gallows, or black, humor. Robinson (1991) notes, "Black humor is a defense against the horror, against whatever it is we fear, and is a way to master it and give us a sense of control by laughing at it" (p. 81). For healthcare staff, humor is a way of distancing oneself from the patient or the situation. Gallows humor allows the provider to continue giving compassionate care because it releases tension. Robinson (1991) notes that joking among staff members does not interfere with their ability to care. In fact, it actually adds to the quality of performance because of the reduced perceived emotional stress. One caution is needed, however. Gallows humor must be used judiciously. It can be hurtful if the wrong person overhears it.

Playing jokes on each other is one way healthcare workers can use humor to alleviate stress. Here are two examples of practical jokes:

- In one hospital the nurses on the day shift would sometimes make an old woman out of pillows in an empty bed for the night nurse, with all the appropriate papers in a file (Astedt-Kurki & Isola, 2001).

- One of the LPNs came into the staff development office where Annie, the CPR mannequin, was being cleaned after a CPR class. She took Annie and carefully placed her on the toilet seat in the private bath of the office. The next person to enter the bathroom was the nursing director. The nursing director immediately turned around and said to the LPN, "Ms. P., you're at it again," at which point those in the office started laughing (personal experience).

Teamwork is an important aspect of providing effective health care. Humor helps foster an atmosphere of teamwork. According to Robinson (1991), one intensive care unit that had no staff turnover in 7 years reported that the climate of humor was one factor in the productivity and effectiveness of the group. Without humor, work would be colorless and devoid of enjoyment.

Kinde (2002) offers a suggestion for helping nurses build humor into the workplace. These ideas can be incorporated by all healthcare providers. He suggests taking a comment that someone makes and creating a "shopping list" of events. The example he uses is to take a comment such as "This place is a war zone" and make two separate lists. One list can be called "hospital things" and the other can be called "military things." The next step is to brainstorm by making the lists as long as possible. Everyone can take part in the development of the list. The last step is to create humorous connections between the two lists.

Kinde (2002) shares his list of "Ten Ways a Hospital is Like the Military." Table 4-1 highlights excerpts from this list.

TABLE 4-1: BUILDING WORKPLACE HUMOR

Excerpts from "Ten Ways a Hospital is Like the Military."

- In the military, soldiers take orders from people with silver and gold on their shoulders. In a hospital, nurses take orders from people with silver and gold in their wallets.

- When discharged from the hospital after a lower GI series, you get the GI bill.

- Nurses, like soldiers, see a lot of privates.

- Nurse training is like boot camp. Never before had you seen so many bald body parts.

- In the military, a fatigue is what you wear. In nursing, it's what wears on you.

(Kinde, 2002. p. 24)

USING HUMOR WITH PATIENTS

Humor helps healthcare providers connect with their patients. You say you are not one to tell jokes because you never remember the punch line? Have no fear, jokes are not the only way to use humor with patients. Humor can sometimes be found in an off-hand remark that comes out funny. Sometimes it is deliberate. Other times, humor involves recognizing a humorous attempt by a patient.

The Iowa Intervention Project has identified at least 357 nursing intervention classifications (NIC). One of these is humor. The operational definition of humor given to this NIC is, "Facilitating the patient to perceive, appreciate and express what is funny, amusing or ludicrous in order to establish relationships, relieve tension, release anger, facilitate learning or cope with painful feelings" (Wooten, 1996, p. 47).

A study by Adamle (2001) found that humor in hospice settings was more often initiated by the patient than the healthcare provider. Humor gives patients an alternate way of looking at their situation and helps them explore new coping skills and gain some element of control (Bellert, 1989).

A study by Lippert (2001), which investigated the use of humor in a long-term care setting, found

> The nurse went in to check her respiratory distress patient in the Critical Care Unit who was getting oxygen via a mask.
>
> The nurse tried to talk to him, but all she could get out of him was gasping and unintelligible talk.
>
> Finally, the nurse thrust a note pad and pencil at the patient and said, "I can't understand you, sir. Please write it down."
>
> The patient weakly scribbled on the pad, "Get your foot off my oxygen tube!"
>
> *Note.* From NursingHumor.com. Used with permission.

that humor was more often initiated by staff in this setting. The humorous exchanges tended to occur during care tasks or routine rituals, such as medication passes or meals. The most common type of humor used was conversational humor. Even with patients who have dementia, the use of humor, and especially the response of laughter, helps form a connection between patients and staff.

Through analysis of nurses' diaries, Astedt-Kurkie and Isola (2001) found that humor could be initiated by the nurse *and* the patient. Because observation was not a part of this study, it is difficult to know who was more likely to initiate the humor. However, humor seemed to help nurses and patients deal with routine care, unpleasant procedures, embarrassing events, and difficult situations. Humor also functioned as a way for people to admit that they did not know everything without "losing face" (Astedt-Kurkie & Isola, 2001, p. 457).

In reviewing these studies, a question arises: Does the setting influence who initiates the humor? In Adamle's (2001) study, did the nurses hold back and wait to see if the patient would use humor because the nurses were dealing with patients who were dying? Were the nurses demonstrating caution and respect for their patient's needs and emotional status? In Lippert's (2001) study, did the nurses initiate humor because it was a situation in which a rapport had been established and the social norm allowed nurses to feel comfortable with using humor? These questions raise issues for further study and further thought by nurses and other healthcare providers. When is it appropriate to use humor? How can healthcare providers know when humor will be appropriate and appreciated? Sometimes they do not, and humor might be used inappropriately. In this situation, the provider must be sensitive enough to recognize it and apologize.

Humor can help establish rapport with a patient, or it can help enhance an established rapport. It is important to note that the healthcare provider needs to be sensitive to a patient's emotional state if she or he is going to be the initiator of humor. Sometimes patients may prefer to be the initiators of humor. Another concern is that ill-timed humor can be hurtful.

Establishing a level of rapport may be necessary for humor to be an effective method of communicating, especially in situations where the patient is in therapy. In the following situation, the patient had been working with a therapist to deal with her depression and substance abuse. This woman was inclined to blame herself for everything occurring within her family and extended family. This woman found it difficult to find any humor in any of life's events. During the session she blamed herself for her children's difficulty with learning. When the therapist said, "Let me understand this, you have caused them to be unable to do their homework. Have you broken their arms, not paid the electricity bills, or played loud music in order to distract them?" she missed the irony of the statement. Taking the comment seriously she said she had not done any of that. She goes on to explain that she perceives the children are unhappy to have her for a mother and that her "whole family blames me for everything," including that her brothers do not talk to each other and that her mother is ill. The counselor continued.

Counselor: Have you been watching television lately? The president just went on TV to discuss the economy. I should think that he would have mentioned you directly.

Patient: What do you mean by that?

Counselor: Well, it seems to me that you blame yourself, hold yourself accountable for everything. Have you considered attributing any inflation worries or depressed economy, or global warming, or increased terrorist activities all to you? I'm surprised that you left those out.

Patient: (For the first time appreciating the humor in the question – she began to laugh and her facial expression freed up.) I guess you are right. I do tend to blame myself for everything. (Goldin & Bordan, 1999, p. 408).

One thing students of healthcare programs, whether it be nursing, social work, counseling, or medical school, are commonly cautioned about is offering too much self-disclosure. Humor is one method of self-disclosure that can help build a bond in a way that is not threatening to the provider. For example, a healthcare worker can share with a patient or client a situation similar to the one the person is dealing with but with a humorous overtone. This communication can help the individual put his or her situation into perspective without threat.

Personal Insight

I am a cancer survivor and a firm believer in the use of humor as a coping mechanism. It is not uncommon for someone to refer a patient with breast cancer to me. One of the things I do is share my own struggle – including the ups and downs of dealing with a potentially life-threatening disease. I also share my strong belief that humor works as an effective coping mechanism, and that I now sport a smiley face on my reconstructed breast. A number of patients have shared how helpful it was to look at the lighter side of breast cancer and how the conversation reminded them to find the humor in their own situations.

Humor can be used to ask questions about sensitive subjects, such as dying, sexuality, loss of control, and suicide. "Humor becomes the 'how' of asking and laughter becomes the language of closeness" (Gullickson, 1995). As noted by Adamle (2001), even during the terminal phase of life, humor serves as a means of allowing the patient, the family, and the nurse to view the patient as still possessing life.

This need to still be viewed as being alive is apparent in the following interchange between a nurse and a hospice patient. The patient was an elderly gentleman who was an avid fisherman. He was admitted to hospice with metastatic colon cancer and was in a lot of pain. On one of the visits, the nurse asked, "How have you been feeling? Anxious at all?" The following discussion ensued (Adamle, 2001, p. 117):

Patient: I am anxious to get the boat out, anxious to have warmer weather, anxious to drop my line in the lake, anxious to catch my first fish this year! Next week you'll have to do your visit down at the lake 'cause I'll be there!

Family: I'll drive her down there to see you. (rolls her eyes and laughs)

Nurse: That's a deal! (laughs)

Dementia is a concern for many people as they age. The following interchange took place between a hospice nurse and a 71-year-old female who was living in a nursing home (Adamle, 2001, p. 117):

Nurse: I have to write this down (vital signs). I'm getting so forgetful. If I don't write it down, I'll lose track of what I'm doing! (laughs and holds her head in her hands)

Patient: Oh please, don't talk to me about that, honey. (laughs) Just you wait until you are my age and in my shape! (laughs)

Humor can also work to decrease a stressful situation, as in the continued exchange with the above patient. When the nurse asked if the patient had any new problems the nurse should know about, the patient recounted a story of being left on the bedpan. She put her light on and no one came, so the patient called the front desk on her personal phone and asked if someone could get her off the pan or if she should call 911 (Adamle, 2001, p. 118).

I used humor to cope with emotions that defied words following my mastectomy and reconstructive surgery. I explain it this way:

It was the second night after surgery and I needed to go to the bathroom. Being the "good nurse," I got out of bed, unplugged my IV pump, and got into the bathroom. Because I had a TRAM flap, I was unable to comfortably put my feet on the floor, so I pulled up the shower seat, rested my feet on the rung of the seat, and was sitting there trying to void when the tears started. I cried and cried, and suddenly I thought, if anyone comes in right now and sees me, I will look so ridiculous. At that, I started to laugh at the absurdity of the situation.

The ability to laugh at the situation, to see the funny side of a situation that was difficult, helped me get through that particular event and the night. It helped make the situation seem less distressing. Today, it serves as a piece of information that can be shared.

At a humor conference, a well-known humor presenter was sharing an experience he had when he was asked to talk to a group of patients with cancer. He wanted to make sure that the group leader understood that he was a humorist and that he talked about humor. He wondered if humor would be an appropriate topic for people dealing with cancer. The group leader reassured him that he knew that the presenter talked about humor and that was why he had been asked to present. As the group began, the presenter became concerned. The group members sat in a circle, and each person shared a little about his or her story. As the gravity of the disease processes were shared, the presenter prayed that God would reveal some way of presenting his material without seeming inappropriate. Finally, one man said, "I was diagnosed with cancer and told I had about 6 months to live, so I gave away all my winter clothes, but I have lived long enough to see another winter, and I have nothing warm to wear." At that, everyone began to laugh. Finally, the presenter started his presentation. The group was laughing uproariously when a woman stuck her head in the door. "I'm leading a group for bereaved individuals next door," she began. The presenter thought, "Now I've done it." Then she continued, "We would like to know if we can come join you." They joined the group and afterward thanked the presenter for a chance to be able to laugh.

Nurses are commonly taught the proper way of administering medications; however, few are taught the proper way to administer humor. Karyn Buxman (Buxman,1996; Gross, Buxman & Ayers, 2009. p. 43), a nurse humorist, talks about the five rights of humor administration. They include the Right Patient, the Right Type of humor, the Right Time, the Right Amount, and the Right Route (Table 4-2).

Dan Gascon (1998) lists 12 things that he says "humor gives where illness lives." According to Gascon, humor

1. helps individuals step back from their illnesses.

2. helps patients gain perspective.

3. shows patients that there is more to life than just physical disabilities.

4. opens minds to realities that are fun, joyous, and light.

5. makes people smile.

6. achieves states that are tranquil, flowing, and worry-free.

7. validates that, although a person may be seriously ill or in the process of dying, at the moment, they are alive.

8. involves everyone in conversation.

9. insulates against loneliness and fear.

10. is a sign of approval, caring, compassion, and connection.

11. loves them with lightness and joy.

12. lifts the spirit and speeds recovery.

(Gascon, 1998, p. 5)

USING HUMOR WITH DYING PATIENTS

I'm not afraid to die, I just don't want to be there when it happens.

– Woody Allen

As previously noted, humor is appropriate for use with patients who are dying. In most cases, dying people still want to be a part of life for as long as they can. As Alan Klein (1998) stated in his book *The Courage to Laugh,* which shares anecdotal stories about humor in the face of death and dying, "[Humor] is nature's way of giving us a perspective on a situation and allowing us to rise above it. Humor helps us keep our balance when life throws us a curve ball" (p. 4)

There is nothing funny about dying or the grief of impending loss of a loved one. However, funny things happen as a person dies. It is up to those involved in the situation to decide whether they want to see the humor. Remember, however, that what might be humorous to one person may not be to

TABLE 4-2: THE FIVE RIGHTS OF HUMOR ADMINISTRATION	
Right Patient	For some patients, humor is inappropriate or unhelpful. Some patients do not appreciate humor.
Right Type	At times, certain types of humor, such as gallows or black humor, may be in poor taste. Sarcastic humor aimed at the patient in the form of a put-down is also inappropriate.
Right Time	Timing is crucial. Humor might be appropriate with patients who have mild to moderate anxiety but inappropriate during a crisis or when the anxiety level of the patient is high. At times of high anxiety, humor may be distracting and offensive.
Right Amount	Too much of a good thing ruins effectiveness. Continued attempts at joking and humor may be overwhelming and annoying.
Right Route	Humor does not have to come in the form of jokes. In some cases, being able to laugh at oneself or the situation is most effective. Spontaneous humor is often appreciated more than joke telling.

(Buxman, 1996; Gross, Buxman, & Ayers, 2009, p. 43.)

another. Humor can be hurtful or inappropriate. However, as noted earlier, humor can also be helpful and appreciated. For example, one patient responded to humor with the comment, "I'm so tired of everyone being so solemn. It is great to be able to laugh."

Certain barriers make the use of humor during death and dying uncommon. These barriers include

- the American cultural view that death is a negative experience to be feared;

- the belief that dying people should be approached with a muted display of positive emotions (Herth, 1995);

- the physical, emotional, and social pain and loss that dying evokes;

- the physical deterioration that affects dying people and, in return, affects all those connected with them.

A descriptive study by Herth (1995) involving 14 terminally ill adults indicated that sharing positive feelings helped the participants feel "like a real person again" (p. 220). The positive effects of humor as seen by these participants are as follows:

- It helped maintain a sense of belonging.

- It promoted relaxation.

- It helped alter perceptions.

- It offered a feeling of warmth, a sense of light-heartedness, and delight.

- Occasionally, it offered hearty laughter.

- It was a "life-enricher" and a "life-enhancer."

One patient who had been incontinent shared how she really appreciated the nurse's aide's comment when she shared her embarrassment. The aide looked at her and said, "Don't worry. What goes in must come out." The two of them had a little laugh together and it broke the tension.

Another patient who was in the intensive care unit had a monitor that kept going off. The nurse was getting frustrated, but the patient looked at her and said, "Don't worry, if I can hear it I'm still alive."

USING HUMOR WITH FAMILY CAREGIVERS

Humor can help the healthcare provider connect with a patient's significant others. Remember that appropriate humor can be a good means of communication. It can break down barriers and relieve tension. Caregivers may feel powerlessness, fear, frustration, anxiety, or any number of negative emotions when a loved one is ill. The use of humor can assist the caregiver in dealing with all of these emotions. It can sometimes be hard to see the humor in a situation, and the caregiver might need a little assistance. Other times, humor is inappropriate. The nurse needs to be sensitive to the appropriateness and timing of humor.

When a situation seems to be grave, the use of humor may be inappropriate. However, humor may also be a way of lightening up a situation. For example, when my husband was dying, humor was an appropriate tool to lessen the anticipatory grief. However, ill-timed humor might have been hurtful. Being alert to patient and caregiver needs allows a care provider to help the patient and the family during a difficult time. An example of this occurred with the 70-year-old avid fisherman mentioned earlier. During a revisit, the nurse asked about anxiety:

Nurse: How have you been feeling? Anxious at all?

Wife: Which one of us? (laughs)

This exchange could be a good opportunity for the nurse to explore the family members' level of anxiety. Awareness of the underlying messages behind the humor can allow the nurse to design interventions useful to the patient and family.

Family members may use humor as a means of helping the healthcare provider as well. After my husband died, the doctor who admitted him came onto the unit. I could see that the doctor was shaken by the death, and he confirmed this when he said, "This should never have happened. We should have been able to turn around his idiopathic thrombocytopenia." Feeling that I needed to do something for both the doctor and myself, I said: "If he had lived, he would have had one problem after another; then he would have gotten depressed, and then I would have had to kill him. So he saved me from going to jail." At that, the doctor and I chuckled, and the tension of us two grievers decreased.

HUMOR ASSESSMENT

Nurses are always doing assessments of different body systems and mental capacities. Counselors and psychologists are always doing mental status assessments. What about doing a humor assessment? The humor assessment helps to discover the type of humor patients use or appreciate as a means of designing humor interventions appropriate for the patient. Table 4-3 includes some questions that can be asked. These are only suggested questions. It is up to each care provider to decide which questions and how many are appropriate for a particular patient.

Part of a humor assessment involves being cognitively aware of the patient's response to humor. Does the patient smile or laugh at lighthearted remarks? Does the patient watch sitcoms on television? Does the patient seem to use humor as an avoidance or defense mechanism? Because humor can be used inappropriately to avoid problem solving or dealing with feelings, the healthcare provider must assess the possibility that the patient is using defensive humor, which might interfere with coping.

TABLE 4-3: HUMOR ASSESSMENT QUESTIONS

- What importance does humor play in your life?
- What makes you laugh?
- Who makes you laugh?
- Since your illness, do you find yourself using humor more, less, or about the same?
- What is one area of your life to which you would like to add humor?
- Do you consider humor a source of relaxation?
- What kind of jokes do you like?
- What does the phrase "laughter is the best medicine" mean to you?
- What type of humor offends you?
- What is your favorite sitcom? What is it about that show that makes you laugh?

THE NEGATIVE SIDE OF HUMOR

As previously mentioned, humor can have negative effects. This section explores some of the inappropriate uses of humor. Harvey (1998) discusses a 1956 study by Levine, who found that there are three possible responses to humor:

1. It evokes no anxiety and, therefore, the listener responds with indifference.

2. It evokes and then immediately dissipates anxiety. The listener considers the humor amusing or funny.

3. It arouses anxiety without decreasing it. The listener does not find the humor funny and may even feel disgust or embarrassment.

One type of humor that can be destructive is hostile humor. Examples of hostile humor include cultural slurs or comments about a person's behavior. Hostile humor may also be used to help express anger, such as the patient who wanted to know if she should call 911 in order to be removed from the bedpan. However, if the patient's nurse was tired and frustrated, she may not have seen the humor in this comment. Here is another example: An alert patient broke her leg while on vacation. She was admitted to a nursing home for rehabilitation but was unable to get out of bed without assistance. Her roommate, a resident with dementia, was trying to get out of bed to go to the bathroom. The patient put on her call light but no one came. She called for help and still no one came. Fearful that her roommate would fall and injure herself, the patient started throwing things against the wall to make noise until the aide came in. Instead of seeing the humor in the situation, the aide told the woman that her behavior was inappropriate. In telling the story to the nurse the next day, the resident and the nurse had a good laugh.

Some gallows humor can be hurtful or offensive to others. The term "GOMER" is one example of this type of gallows humor. Short for "Get Out of My Emergency Room," GOMER was coined by Dr. Samuel Shem, who wrote a "hilarious and often heart-rending book called *House of God*" (Wooten, 1996, p. 25). The term was originally used to refer to patients who were very ill, uncooperative, unappreciative of help, or confused but is now commonly used to describe patients who are in a vegetative state. Although gallows humor can help care providers deal with difficult events and situations, it can have a negative effect on the people to whom it is directed and can lead to insult and alienation (Harvey, 1998).

Humor is sometimes used to avoid the therapeutic process or avoid painful issues. This may take the form of "scapegoating," or aiming the humor at one person in the group. This use of humor can be hurtful and nonproductive. Humor is also inappropriate if the receiver of the message does not know whether the speaker is serious or joking.

When using humor it is important for healthcare providers to be aware of their own emotions. Humor can be a left-handed way of expressing anger or aggression, which is something the care provider does not want to impart on the patient. The care provider needs to be cautious and avoid giving the patient a feeling that they are not being taken seriously.

If a health professional has doubts about how another person might receive a joke, it is best not to tell it. Humor used with patients should always be a way to facilitate, not interrupt the healing process. Before saying something that might be hurtful, the person should think about how he or she might feel in a similar situation. It is one thing for an individual who has a disability to make a joke about the disability. This type of self-effacing humor might help relieve tension. However, if an able-bodied person makes the same joke, the comment might be considered a slur.

STORIES FROM THE FIELD

The following examples illustrate how humor has been used to help people deal with illness or hospitalization.

Bob, a man in his 50s, had a tumor on his knee that required surgery. Being aware of the power of laughter in the healing process, the patient asked Annette Goodheart, a laughter therapist, to visit him right after surgery. He had a large 10-in. to 12-in. suture around his knee, but his knee was wrapped in such a manner that he was able to remove a portion of the outer bandage. Dr. Goodheart had him gently press around the incision area and say, "Ow!" A pillow was ready so that if a big "Ow!" came out, the patient could stifle the sound and not alarm the hospital staff.

As he pressed around the incision and said "Ow," he laughed. The more he pressed and the more he said "Ow," the more he laughed. In between the laughter, he related the events of the surgery. By processing the emotions that occurred during surgery, he prevented tension from storing around the traumatized area, allowing his body's healing mechanisms to function faster and more freely.

After about half an hour, the patient was able to endure more and more pressure without feeling pain. At this point, the surgeon came in to see how the patient was doing. He came toward the bed and said, "Bob, how are you feeling?" Bob kicked out his leg. The surgeon was so shocked, he almost fell over backward. Bob was on his feet within several hours, walking around the hall. He reported that the surgeon was astounded by the rate of his recovery. (Goodheart, 1994, p. 59-60)

The following story came from personal communication with an acquaintance:

"Personally, I am not naturally inclined to see humor in things and tend to be too serious. It always takes me longer to get a joke. Recently, my cage has been rattled to give me a wake-up call. Surgery for a skin graft in January left me with unhappy results of the loss of 60% of the graft. After trying everything medically possible, along with prayer, a friend suggested I try humor. I now intentionally factor in times of watching comedy and laughing every day. The graft is healing, and a really neat benefit of more wholesome relationships with my family has resulted."

The following story was received via e-mail.

An old man often sat at a specific corner table with his friends. He rarely went more than 10 or 15 minutes without laughing. When asked how he managed to stay in such a wonderful mood all the time, he responded that his laughter did not always mean he was in a good mood. He explained that he laughed for two reasons. One was to get into a good mood. He lived alone and did not like it. He knew that laughter would lift his spirits, so he forced himself to laugh until he really was feeling good. The other reason was that he had arthritis and had a lot of aches and pains. One day he and his friends were doubling up with laughter about

pranks they had played when they were kids. He discovered that his arthritis pain had disappeared during the laughter and did not show up again until an hour later. From that day on, he was a laugher. It was his way of managing pain and taking control in a way that improved his quality of life.

Being able to find humor in different situations is important. The following are stories that nurses have shared about funny things that have happened at work.

I was admitting a patient one night and asking the usual questions on the admit form. When I asked my patient if she had any allergies, she informed me that she was allergic to Ipecac. Seems it made her throw up every time she took it. – H. Sox

When I worked in traumatic brain injury rehabilitation, a nurse briefly placed a bisacodyl suppository at a patient's bedside. He promptly ate it.

We called the local poison control center hotline to find out what to do. After listening to our story, the nurse at the hotline reassured us. She said, "This, too, will pass." – K. Dunn

One day in the OR, I was holding a patient in a sitting position while the anesthesiologist was administering a spinal anesthetic for a TURP. Warning the patient of the impending injection, the physician said, "Little prick here!"

The patient, who was bending over, staring at his crotch, said, "Yeah, I know. It's been that way all my life." – M. Wren

SUMMARY

Humor is an important part of health care. The anecdotal stories in this chapter present a personal picture from nurses' and patients' views of the effectiveness of humor in the healthcare setting. These stories present a colorful picture of how humor can be effective for the patient and the nurse. Studies show that humor helps patients deal with the difficulties of illness and helps form a connection between nurse and patient. Some studies have explored who commonly initiates humor in the healthcare setting – sometimes it is the nurse and sometimes it is the patient. Deciding when it is appropriate to use humor can be challenging. Rapport and sensitivity are keys in deciding if humor is appropriate. Humor initiated by the patient is commonly a clue that humor is an acceptable response. However, it is important to remember that, although humor can be healing and form a connection between people, it can also be hurtful. Being sensitive, alert to when humor might be helpful, and spontaneous is important.

The most important lessons from this chapter are:

1. Remember the Five Rights of Humor Administration
   - The Right Patient
   - The Right Type
   - The Right Time
   - The Right Amount
   - The Right Route
2. Look for humorous situations to help lighten yourself.
3. Be alert for when humor might be used as a cover-up for feelings or thoughts that should be addressed.

EXAM QUESTIONS

CHAPTER 4
Questions 28-35

Note: Choose the one option that BEST answers each question.

28. According to Buxman, the three main functions of humor in health care are

    a. psychological, social, spiritual.
    b. spiritual, social, communication.
    c. psychological, social, communication.
    d. focal, psychological, social.

29. One appropriate way to diffuse tension at work is to

    a. scream.
    b. share a joke.
    c. mumble to yourself.
    d. throw something.

30. A common form of humor between nurses in high-stress areas such as the emergency room is

    a. incongruent-resolution humor.
    b. illusion formation.
    c. gallows humor.
    d. comical wordplay.

31. A patient who recently sustained an injury that left her paraplegic states with a laugh, "I guess I won't be needing those high heels I just bought." The nurse should recognize that the patient

    a. has overreacted to her paraplegia.
    b. is angry about the money she spent.
    c. is using humor to cope with painful feelings.
    d. wants to give her shoes to the nurse.

32. A patient is admitted for same day surgery. The nurse notices that the patient seems very anxious. A good approach that might decrease the patient's anxiety and open the door for exploring the reason behind the anxiety is

    a. after introductions, hand the patient the hospital gown and state, "Please put on our Paris original."
    b. state, "Why are you so anxious? It's only a small surgery."
    c. start talking about the type of surgery the patient is scheduled for, and its complications.
    d. ignore the patient's behavior and, in a very professional manner, go through the admission procedures.

33. The study by Adamle that looked at humor in the hospice setting discovered that humor was initiated most often by

    a. the nurse.
    b. the patient.
    c. the family.
    d. the nurse's aide.

34. The purpose of a humor assessment is to

    a. discover what jokes the patient already knows.
    b. get the patient thinking about using humor to cope.
    c. prove that patients use humor.
    d. discover the type of humor that might be appropriate for the patient.

35. *A nurse is admitting a Jewish woman to the hospital. The woman is wearing designer clothes. To establish rapport, the nurse tells an ethnic joke about a Jewish princess. Instead of laughing, the patient looks offended. Later, the nurse overhears the patient tell the same joke to a Jewish friend, who laughs at the joke.*

The difference between the patient's two responses is best explained by

a. the patient thinking she missed something because she did not see anything funny in the joke, so she decided to see how her friend reacted.

b. the patient did not understand the joke and hoped her friend could explain it to her.

c. the patient was too nervous to appreciate the humor at the time of admission.

d. the tendency for self-effacing humor is better accepted by the receiver when it is shared with others of the same ethnic or situational group.

CHAPTER 5

THE PSYCHOBIOLOGY OF HUMOR AND LAUGHTER

CHAPTER OBJECTIVE

After completing this chapter the reader will be able to recognize the psychobiological effects of humor.

LEARNING OBJECTIVES

After studying this chapter, the reader will be able to

1. describe the cognitive factors in humor perception.

2. explain the neurobiological process by which someone "gets the joke."

3. describe the process of laughter.

4. discuss the possible causes of pathological laughter.

INTRODUCTION

If you lose the power to laugh, you lose the power to think.

– Clarence Seward Darrow

Have you ever wondered how we understand humor? How does our brain process the information and recognize that something funny has occurred? What is it about a joke that causes us to laugh? Researchers have studied how the brain processes information that tells a person that something comical or funny has occurred. Exploring the neuropsychology of humor helps us understand the process by which a person comprehends a joke. Researchers have been able to visualize brain regions involved in a wide range of psychological responses, including humor through the use of functional magnetic resonance imaging (fMRI) and other neuroimaging techniques (Martin, 2007). An fMRI offers high resolution, noninvasive reports of neural activity. This neural activity is detected by a blood oxygen level–dependent signal that allows the researcher to see the process as it is happening.

This chapter takes a serious look at the process of "getting the joke" and appreciating the humorous. It will explore what we know about the cognitive process of laughter by looking at how the brain responds when we laugh.

Human laughter has a recognizable sound no matter from what part of the world a person originates (Gervais & Wilson, 2005). We will look at the nature of laughter and how we produce the sounds that are recognized as laughter. The chapter will also explore pathological laughter as a way of alerting healthcare providers to be sensitive to laughter that does not seem to be a response to mirth. Pathological laughter could signal a brain dysfunction or mental illness requiring medical attention.

Cognition and Humor

The brain is an amazing organ with many functions. One of these functions is the ability to process information. In Chapter 1 we looked at the different theories of humor. These theories related to how one perceives humor and understands that something funny has happened. Humor perception and humor comprehension tend to be used synonymously in the literature. Ziv (1984) denotes a distinction between these aspects of humor. Ziv sees humor comprehension as the ability to perceive relationships or ideas in incongruous ways, and humor appreciation is viewed as the ability to understand and feel pleasure from humorous messages. In other words, humor comprehension occurs when we "get the joke," and humor appreciation occurs when we experience an element of enjoyment from the humorous material.

In order to understand a joke we need to have some knowledge of the material or information to recognize the incongruity and the resolution. Brain studies were done via neuroimaging while subjects read or were presented with jokes, humorous material, and non-humorous material. These imaging studies have increased neurosciences knowledge of the areas of the brain that become active while attempting to process the information presented. These studies look at the process of working memory (Uekermann, Daum & Channon, 2007). Working memory is a cognitive psychology theoretical construct referring to structures and processes that temporarily store and manipulate information. It is believed that prior social and cultural knowledge acquired during childhood and adolescence leads to enhanced ability to access relevant information in working memory for joke comprehension.

In an interview for *Humor & Health Letter* (Humor in the brain, 1995), Dr. Peter Derks, Professor of Psychology at the College of William and Mary, shared the following information:

- Changes occurring in the brain when a person really laughs at an event he or she finds funny are different than those occurring when reading a joke that does not elicit laughter. This difference might relate to some kind of releaser process. This electric response in the brain may stimulate the endocrine responses that Berk and colleagues found in their studies. (Information on these changes can be found in the chapter on physiological changes.)

- Response to humor involves both of the brain's hemispheres. The left hemisphere (the one involved with language) sets up the joke. The right hemisphere (the one involved in pattern recognition and processing simultaneous information) is activated when we "get the joke."

- When a person reads a joke, the left hemisphere of the brain is active. The response, however, instantaneously activates the entire cortex. Derks states, "As the process continues, the left hemisphere begins to shut down, and the right picks up. Then both hemispheres join in a sort of holistic dance" (p. 26).

- Humor involves the whole person and all information processing abilities – cognition, emotion, feelings, and ideas.

THE BRAIN'S RESPONSE TO HUMOR

A number of studies indicate that humor comprehension may require different underlying cognitive abilities (Baldwin, 2007). Some studies have explored how people with brain injury or damage from the stroke process react to subtle information, such as that found in humor (Baldwin, 2007; Cheang & Pell, 2006; Martin, 2007). It has been noted that individuals with right frontal damage appear to have the greatest difficulty with tasks demonstrating humor appreciation, although this was not the case when the participants were requested to finish the last line of a joke (Cheang &

Pell, 2006). When asked to finish the last line of a joke, individuals with right hemisphere damage (RHD) tended to choose slapstick endings, even if the ending did not correlate to the joke. This finding indicated an understanding that a surprise element is what can make something seem humorous, although they were unable to accurately choose which surprising element was coherent with the text of the joke.

An example of the joke completion task follows:

Mable walked into a pastry shop. After surveying all the pastries, she decided on a chocolate pie. "I'll take that one," Mable said to the attendant, "the whole thing." The attendant asked, "Shall I cut it in four or eight pieces?"

   a.   Mabel said, "Well, there are five people for dessert tonight, so eight pieces would be about right."

   b.   Mable said, "You make the most delicious sweet rolls in town."

   c.   Then the attendant squirted whipped cream in Mable's face.

   d.   Mable said, "Four pieces please. I'm on a diet."

The response those with RHD were most likely to choose was **c**, the slapstick response. The expected, or correct response for the joke completion task was **d**.

Studies of individuals with brain lesions indicated interesting aspects concerning the processing of information (Uekerman et al., 2007). These studies were conducted using incongruity theory as the basis for investigation. Individuals with lesions to the right hemisphere demonstrated significant impairment in distinguishing the correct punch line to joke completion tasks, as noted above. Individuals who had left hemisphere damage tended to choose responses that were straight forward (which would be response **a** in the example above). Uekermann et al. (2007) note that this indicates that left hemisphere damaged patients are

"impaired at the first stage (incongruity detection)" and right hemisphere damaged individuals were impaired "at the second stage (resolution)" (p. 556). Other studies discussed indicate that people with damage to the right frontal lobes were not able to detect differences between funny and neutral verbal comments and usually selected slapstick endings on joke completion tests. The results of these studies indicate that the right frontal lobes of the brain might be one of the main regions in humor processing.

Another chance to explore brain-driven laughter occurred at the University of California at Los Angeles (UCLA) Medical Center with a young, seizure-prone woman (Strubbe, 2003). When a restricted area of the woman's left frontal cortex was electrically stimulated, she laughed consistently and perceived whatever she was looking at as funny. Low levels of stimulation made her smile. Higher levels of stimulation lead to belly laughter. Perhaps the future will provide more information on the physiological effects of laughter and the use of methods other than medication to decrease depression.

Strubbe (2003) explains that, although the left side understands puns, complex non-word play jokes are processed by the right-side gyri, which then triggers activity in other parts of the brain. Doskoch (1996) notes that about "four-tenths of a second after we hear the punch line of a joke – but before we laugh – a negatively charged wave of electricity sweeps through the cortex"(p. 3). This electrical wave, which can be seen on an EEG, eventually covers the entire cerebral cortex. The brain's response to laughter differs from emotional responses in that emotional responses are mainly the function of the frontal lobe, whereas laughter occurs in the left, front, right, and rear of the cerebral cortex as well as in the motor section of the brain.

Figure 5-1 demonstrates the areas of the brain that we have a good idea are stimulated by humor and laughter.

FIGURE 5-1: BRAIN REGIONS INVOLVED IN EMOTIONAL AND COGNITIVE FACTORS OF HUMOR AND LAUGHTER

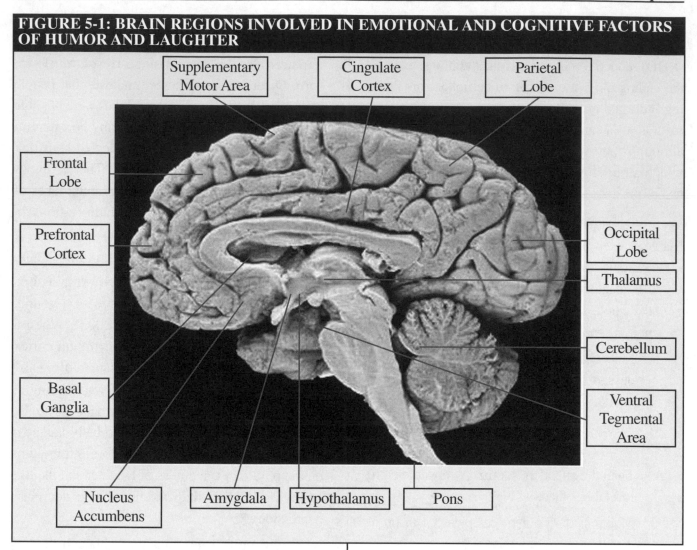

BIOLOGY OF LAUGHTER

I am thankful for laughter, except when milk comes out of my nose.

– Woody Allen

Laughter is a way of communicating to another individual that one is feeling a certain emotion. In many cases laughter expresses the emotion of mirth. It may, however, express other emotions, such as nervousness, fear, or disgust. For the purpose of this text, the main emphasis will be on laughter as an expression of mirth.

In his text, *The Psychology of Humor: An Integrative Approach,* Martin (2007) discusses Charles Darwin's comment that laughter appears to be essentially an emotional expression, which is "one of the largely hardwired behavior patterns"

that humans use to communicate many positive or negative emotions (p. 155). The movement of the mouth while smiling and laughing appears to have different evolutionary origins. However, they are closely related and occur on a continuum of emotional intensity (Martin, 2007). We know that the same muscles are involved with smiling and laughing, with stronger contractions of longer duration occurring with laughter.

What do we know about the sounds of laughter? We know that they are distinct sounds, and that there seems to be a quality of contagiousness. It is hard not to laugh when you are in the presence of someone who is laughing. Robert Provine (2000a) a neuroscientist at the University of Maryland, decided he wanted to "crack the laugh code" (p. 56). To attempt to satisfy his curiosity, he recorded

51 different people laughing. He then took these recordings and, along with an undergraduate student, Yvonne Young, analyzed the sounds using a sound analyzer that generated a detailed graphic and numerical description of the sound frequencies and amplitudes. In the beginning, people found it difficult to laugh on command, probably because they were not feeling the emotion of mirth. However, through viewing the experience as funny, and due to the kidding of the experimenters, they started to laugh spontaneously. It is the spontaneous laughter that was analyzed. They measured the length of the sounds, the number of sounds in succession, and type of sound made, the amplitude (loudness) and the frequency (Hertz) of the sounds.

The sample size used by Provinc was small and subsequently other researchers have recorded and analyzed laughter sounds. Provine (2000a) found that the laughter he recorded was stereotypical in nature. This trend might have been because the people were asked to laugh on demand. Provine (2000a) notes that the sounds we hear connected to laughter are recorded in English as "ha-ha-ha" or "ho-ho-ho" or "he-he-he." They have a certain pattern and rhythm. It is unlikely to hear something that sounds like "ha-ho-ha."

A study conducted by Bachorowski & Owren, (2004) using recordings of 1,024 bouts of laughter from 97 university students, discovered a wide variety of and complexity in acoustical sounds. From this study, Bachorowski & Owren concluded that laughter is a "broad class of sounds with relatively distinct subtypes, each of which function somewhat differently in a social interaction" (p. 1). One way of analyzing sound uses the rate of vibration of the vocal folds, referred to as fundamental frequency (Fo).

The following are the results of their findings:

- Laugh sounds can be grouped into voiced and unvoiced types.

- Voiced laughs have a regular vibration of the vocal cords during expression that gives a tonal, vowel-like sound and are what are thought of as a typical laugh.

- Voiced laughs may have a sing-song quality when the Fo fluctuates in a melodic way over the course of several bursts.

- Unvoiced sounds lack regular vocal-fold vibration resulting in noisy and atonal sounds.

- The sounds could be described as "grunt-like" or "snort-like."

- "Grunt-like" sounds have noise which arises from turbulence in the supralaryngeal vocal tract.

- "Snort-like" sounds originate primarily in the nasal cavities.

- "Many laughs consist of a mix of voiced and unvoiced components." (p. 1)

- Males produced more "grunt-like" laughs.

- Females produced more voiced laughs.

Why study laughter in this detail? Perhaps because it can teach us information about how vocalization occurs, what make laughter contagious so that when one person laughs others will start, or why laughter might be good medicine after surgery or for patients who need to expand their lung capacity.

Regarding lung capacity and laughter, this is what we know from previous research. Laughter usually begins with a forced exhalation, bringing lung volume down to around the normal amount of air remaining after a normal expiration (known as functional residual capacity) (Martin, 2007). This action is followed by a sequence of rapid, repeated, and shallow expirations that sound similar to the "ha-ha-ha" of laughter. By the end of this laugh phase, the lungs reach residual volume, or the amount of the air left in the lung after maximal expiration. As a result, laughter forces out more air from the lungs than would occur during normal breathing. The next action a person takes is to quickly breathe in more air, which fills the lungs again to normal capacity. Because of the amount of expiration, laughter tends to produce a greatly increased breathing volume that could be up to 2.5 times greater than that which occurs during normal breathing.

The diaphragm, abdominal and rib cage muscles that are normally passive during expiration exhibit contractions during the expiratory phase of laughter. Along with the action of these muscles, the larynx becomes involved. The larynx serves as a "valve separating the trachea from the upper aerodigestive tract" (p. 159). The glottis, located in the larynx, initially closes, preventing the air from being exhaled too quickly, and causes a buildup of subglottal air pressure. The glottis then begins to open and close rhythmically, which allows short bursts of pressurized air to escape. When the glottis closes to a narrow slit, the vocal chords will vibrate, and the "ha" sound is produced. The continual movement and changing shape of the glottis while vibrations occur changes the pitch of the laughter's sound during each individual part of the laugh as well as the sound of changing from one laughter phase to another. The sound of the laugh is further influenced by the amount of tension on the vocal chords; the position of the larynx, tongue, and jaw; the shape of the mouth and lips; and the amount of contraction of various facial muscles. All of this is controlled by the person's emotional state. The variation of patterns of phonation and movement from person to person leads to the differences that occur in the sound of each person's laughter (Martin, 2007).

Another way laughter works as a communication signal is through emotional facial display. Ekman and colleagues (cited in Martin, 2007) have identified 18 different smiles. Of all those smiles, only one appears to convey that the person smiling is genuinely enjoying the moment or finds something amusing. Other smiles identified were associated with either forced or fake smiles, or negative emotions such as anxiety or embarrassment mixed with enjoyment. The type of smile indicating genuine enjoyment is called the Duchenne display after the French anatomist who identified it in 1862.

The Duchenne display involves symmetrical, synchronous, and smooth contractions of the zygomatic major and the obicularis oculi muscles of the face. The zygomatic major is the muscle in the cheeks that pulls the lip corners upwards and backwards, whereas the orbicularis oculi is the muscle that surrounds each eye socket and causes wrinkling of the skin at the outer sides of the eyes. (Martin, 2007).

Most types of smiles involve zygomatic major contractions, but only smiles of genuine enjoyment involve the orbicularis oculi. Other muscles may be involved when a person smiles, however the zygomatic and the orbicularis oculi are the only two involved in laughter that is from pure enjoyment. The involvement of other muscles is an indication that other emotions are occurring.

This Duchenne display occurs in laughing as well as in smiling. Laughter often includes other muscles, such as those allowing the mouth to be open and those that lower the jaw. Martin notes that the presence of "crow's feet" wrinkles along the outside of the eyes indicates genuine amusement in smiling and laughing.

A study looking at adults who had lost spouses 6 months previously found a greater frequency of Duchenne laughter significantly correlated with more positive emotions, such as joy and happiness, and less negative emotions, such as guilt, anger, and distress. They later used the videotapes, with the sound off, and had college students rate them on a number of different aspects. The researchers found that the videos displaying more frequent Duchenne laughter evoked higher self-ratings of positive emotions in the observers. The observers also judged the bereaved participants displaying Duchenne laughter as more healthy, better adjusted, more amusing, and less frustrated than those not exhibiting Duchenne display. These findings indicate that the presence of Duchenne display communicates a positive emotion, which in turn, influences the emotional response of the observer (Martin, 2007). Figure 5-2 demonstrates the difference in facial expression between Duchenne and non-Duchenne laughter.

Provine (2004) states, "Laughter is an instinctive, contagious, stereotyped, unconsciously controlled, social play vocalization that is unusual in solitary settings." The issue of laughter being contagious has been an interest for humor scientists for many years. Warren et al. (2006) discovered the area of the brain that is most likely the cause of this contagiousness. Twenty healthy individuals listened to various sounds while having a brain scan using fMRI. These sounds included vomiting, screaming, cheering, laughter, and other positive and negative sounds. All the sounds triggered activity in the brain's premotor cortical region, the area of the brain that prepares the muscles of the face to react according to the stimulus. However, the response was more pronounced when the stimulus was positive. This phenomenon led the researchers to conclude that positive sounds, such as laughter, are more contagious than negative sounds. This information offers one reason that mirroring the behavior of laughter or other positive emotions is more likely to occur than mirroring negative expressions.

Positive emotions such as laughter or cheering are often experienced in group or social situations, such as watching a comedy program or a sports game or enjoying a gathering of friends and colleagues. The brain response to positive emotions primes us to smile or laugh, providing a way to mirror behavior of others, which can help us interact in social situations or with our patients. This knowledge can be helpful in group building situations because projection of positive emotion could play an important part in building strong bonds between people in groups.

Pathological Laughter

Healthcare workers must be alert for laughter that does not seem related to mirth or something humorous, because such laughter may be a key to

FIGURE 5-2: DIFFERENCES IN FACIAL EXPRESSION BETWEEN DUCHENNE AND NON-DUCHENNE LAUGHTER

Spontaneous Duchenne Smile   Intentional Non-Duchenne Smile

Used with permission from Paul Ekman, Ph.D. Retrieved June 3, 2010, from www.paulekman.com.

some type of abnormality in the brain. Although laughter that does not have mirth connected with it is rare in neurosurgical diseases, it does happen. This phenomenon also occurs in some psychological abnormalities. Non-mirth type of laughter may be connected with

- psychological disorders, such as hysteria and schizophrenia;

- pseudobulbar palsy, a disorder affecting muscles that control the tongue, throat, and parts of the face; and

- gelastic epilepsy, a type of epilepsy in which the person has fits of laughter

(Our Ancient Laughing Brain, n.d.).

Pathological laughter has also occurred in brain trauma, demyelinating disorders, vascular accidents, and intracranial tumors, as well as a disease process called trigeminal schwannoma (Jagetia, Kumar, Singh, & Sinha, 2006). Although lesions are uncommon causes of pathological laughter, it can happen, so it is important for healthcare workers to remain alert to that possibility.

The study of patients with abnormalities such as brain lesions has led to the discovery of two separate pathways in the brain that can lead to the physiological production of smiling and laughter (Martin, 2007). One pathway is involuntary and emotional; the other is voluntary and unemotional. Evidence of these separate pathways can be seen in individuals who have had a stroke or other brain injury that affects the voluntary muscles of the face and, therefore, are not able to move their facial muscles but are still able to smile and laugh at something they find funny.

In his text Martin (2007) discusses three categories of pathological laughter mentioned by Duchowny:

1. excessive laughter,

2. forced laughter, and

3. gelastic epilepsy.

Each of these categories has different manifestations and different areas of brain involvement. Conditions of *excessive laughter* encompass heightened feelings of euphoria and amusement, frequent emotional change, inability to inhibit laughter, and lack of insight into the reason for the laughter. This situation is most likely to occur in adulthood, and is often associated with mental disorders such as schizophrenia, mania, and dementia. The part of the brain affected by these disorders is involved in emotional production and regulation, and includes structures in parts of the frontal lobes as well as the limbic system.

Individuals who fit into the *forced laughter* condition have "involuntary outbursts of explosive, self-sustained laughter," which are often accompanied by autonomic disturbances of heart rate, vasomotor control, and sphincter tone" (Martin, 2007, p. 170). They may appear, to others, to be genuinely amused; however, they usually do not feel the positive emotion of mirth that would normally accompany laughter, but instead the experience is unpleasant and embarrassing. These individuals may also have pathological crying with fits of laughter. It might also be difficult to tell if they are crying or laughing. This aspect of laughing and crying indicates that some of the brain centers controlling laughter and crying are located very close together, most likely in that part of the brainstem called the pons. From this condition comes the theory that there is a close link between positive emotions of social play and the distressing emotions of social separation.

The conditions that involve forced laughter usually begin in adulthood and can be caused by a number of degenerate brain conditions such as Parkinson's disease, multiple sclerosis, and amyotrophic lateral sclerosis. Tumors or lesions of the brain related to strokes or brain injury may also cause this type of laughter. Martin notes that there have been some cases in which people have actually laughed themselves to death. It is important for healthcare providers to stay alert to individuals who appear to have labile emotions going from laughing to crying with no apparent reason. It is possible that people with forced laughter may have lesions in many areas of the brain, ranging from the frontal and temporal lobes of the cortex to the ventral mesencephalon, the cerebellum, and the pons.

The last category, gelastic epilepsy, is a rare epileptic condition in which the seizures predominantly take the form of bouts of laughter. These seizures tend to manifest with motor convulsions, abnormal eye movement, and autonomic disturbances. The individual tends to lose consciousness during the seizure and is therefore unaware of the laughter attack. If the individual does not lose consciousness during the seizure, he might report a pleasant feeling of mirth or he may experience the laughter as inappropriate and even unpleasant. The laughter usually lasts less than a minute, but might be prolonged if associated with complex partial seizures. This condition usually starts in childhood. Gelastic epilepsy can even start in infancy, indicating that the neural circuits for laughter are fully developed at birth. This condition is associated with abnormal nonmalignant tissue growth in the hypothalamus. The temporal lobes and the medial frontal lobe also seem to be involved in the seizure activity. Apparently the most common type of gelastic epilepsy is related to a nonmalignant abnormal tissue growth in the hypothalamus (Martin, 2007). From reviewing data related to this epilepsy, it is suggested that the hypothalamus most likely plays an important role in normal laughter as well.

CASE STUDY

A 25-year-old lady presented with uncontrolled laughter of 6 months duration. Her laughter was usually unprovoked and often not associated with mood elevation. The laughter occurred every 15 to 30 minutes and lasted 1 to 2 minutes.

Although she had a depressed mood, the depression was related to concern over her inability to control the laughter. A mini-mental examination demonstrated no psychological pathology. A neurological examination discovered numbness on the left side of her face and left-sided sensorimotor involvement of the trigeminal, facial, and lower cranial nerves. She had some voice changes and difficulty walking.

Questions

1. Would this patient's laughter be considered pathological? Why?

2. Considering her signs and symptoms, what is most likely her problem?

3. What are the chances that depression could be part of the problem and potential cause of the laughter?

4. What steps should the mental health provider take to help this patient?

Discussion

This woman's laughter is definitely pathological, as evidenced by her inability to control the laughter, no mood elevation or feeling of mirth, and the depressed mood associated with her inability to stop laughing. It appears as if the depression is the result of physiological changes, not the cause of them. Plus, her mental status examination demonstrated no psychological pathology. Her physiological condition indicates some brain pathology that might be caused by a lesion. The woman needs a complete neurological examination. It would also be helpful for her to have a counselor work with her to confirm that her laughter is pathological, that she really has not "lost her mind," and to help her through the emotional upheaval she is presently experiencing. One thing that is not needed is to try to teach her appropriate laughter because this present behavior is out of her control.

SUMMARY

Through studying people with pathological laughter and the use fMRIs researchers have been able to track areas of the brain that are affected by laughter. It does appear as if the frontal lobe of the brain is most affected. It also appears that to hear, process, and understand humor both sides of the brain become activated at different times.

Lessons from the chapter include:

- Laughter is contagious (and antibiotics don't help).

- To understand a joke, we have to have some knowledge of the material.

- Ability to understand a joke versus making up a punch line to a joke is probably processed by different parts of the brain, as evidenced by the ability of people with brain injuries to complete a joke task.

- Results of brain imaging studies along with responses from people with brain injuries point to the frontal lobes as being one of the most likely regions for humor processing.

- The left side of the brain hemisphere seems to set up the joke whereas the right side understands the joke.

- Laughter is a form of vocalization that has been recorded and studied.

- The actual trigger of contagiousness of laughter is not known.

- Duchenne laughter is the type of laughter that occurs when something is perceived as funny.

- Specific facial expressions occur with Duchenne laughter, most notably the display of "crow's feet" or those laugh lines women try to cover as they age.

- Three categories have been identified for pathological laughter. They are excessive laughter, forced laughter, and gelastic epilepsy.

EXAM QUESTIONS

CHAPTER 5
Questions 36-43

Note: Choose the one option that BEST answers each question.

36. Working memory is important in humor comprehension because

    a. it allows us to think.

    b. it allows us to access prior information to understand a joke.

    c. this memory helps us to tell the difference between sadness and joy.

    d. it causes the right hemisphere to function.

37. When someone reads a joke, the first part of the brain to be activated is the

    a. right hemisphere, left hemisphere.

    b. cortex, left hemisphere.

    c. pons, right hemisphere.

    d. left hemisphere.

38. The ability to comprehend a joke most likely relies on what brain structure(s)?

    a. the cortex

    b. the brain stem

    c. the skull

    d. the meninges

39. When a person laughs what part of his brain is activated?

    a. Just the left hemisphere.

    b. Only the right hemisphere and motor section.

    c. Only the cortex.

    d. The cortex and motor section.

40. Some people have very distinct laughs. This is dependent on

    a. differences in residual volume.

    b. the way they move their mouth when they laugh.

    c. multiple factors, including vocal chords and facial muscles.

    d. the way a particular person perceives the humor.

41. During a counseling session, the patient starts to laugh at a comment the counselor made. How can the counselor tell if the person was experiencing genuine amusement?

    a. The patient's eyes will have the appearance of "crow's feet."

    b. The patient would be grinning as well as laughing.

    c. The patient will say, "That is really funny."

    d. There will be no contraction of the zygomatic major.

42. During a group session, one of the participants shared a humorous story that resulted in smiles, but when the participant started to laugh as she thought about the event, the other participants started to laugh also. Others tend to laugh when someone laughs because

    a. what was said has to be funny.

    b. the brain's pre-motor cortical region is triggered when someone laughs.

    c. the other participants did not want the person telling the story to feel bad.

    d. politeness is expected in group situations.

43. A patient enters the doctor's office, sits down, picks up a magazine, does not open it, and starts to laugh. The patient has a history of schizophrenia. The laughter lasts about 2 minutes, stops and then a few minutes later starts again. There is no sign of Duchenne display. The most likely reason for this display of laughter is

    a. the patient's psychological disorder.

    b. the patient is anxious.

    c. something on the cover of the magazine was funny.

    d. someone else in the waiting room was laughing.

CHAPTER 6

PSYCHOSOCIAL EFFECTS OF HUMOR

CHAPTER OBJECTIVE

After completing this chapter the reader will be able to discuss the psychosocial effects of humor.

LEARNING OBJECTIVES

After studying this chapter, the reader will be able to

1. describe how humor works as a form of social communication.

2. discuss how humor can be used to handle negative or distressing feelings or events.

3. identify potential gender differences in responses to humor and laughter.

4. discuss the effects of humor in intimate relationships.

5. describe how humor works to relieve stress.

6. discuss the efficacy of humor in bereavement.

HUMOR AS SOCIAL COMMUNICATION

A smile is the shortest distance between two people.
– Victor Borge

Communication is one of the functions of humor. Humor communication is not a formal communication mode, but a casual, indirect form of communication. Humor helps communicate feelings, thoughts, and beliefs to others in a way that might be difficult to convey using other means of communication. Humor can be used to diffuse feelings of anger or impatience by pointing out the absurdity of the situational threat to the ego (Salameh, 1983; Seaward, 1992). Shared humor can help dispel fear and provide a clearer focus on the situation. Humor appears to communicate feelings of fear in a way that diminishes stress in an acceptable manner (Seaward, 1992).

Humor can be an element in effective interpersonal communication (Lippert, 2001). Humor helps dissolve barriers between individuals. As Seaward (1994, cited in Dossey, 1996) noted, "humor has an adhesive quality, which connects and bonds people together, if only for the duration of a joke." Humor can communicate a patient's feelings or concerns that may go beyond words (Gullickson, 1995). If healthcare providers listen to the feelings behind patients' words, therapeutic interventions can be used to help diffuse the tension patients might be feeling. Gullickson (1995) shares an example about a nurse working with a patient about to undergo a kidney transplant. The nurse was preparing the patient for the transplant. When the nurse asked if there was anything the patient wanted to talk about, the patient responded, "Well, you know, it's not like I'm going to die or anything," and then he started to laugh (Gullickson, 1995, p. 20). The nurse had the sense that there were fears behind the attempted humor that were unspeakable. She responded, "You know, I think we need to talk about that" (Gullickson, 1995, p. 21). The nurse's ability to hear the concerns behind the patient's words and laughter, and her comfort in responding to the underlying issues, allowed this patient to discuss his fears and emotional issues that needed attention.

The nurse in the previous example may have realized that laughter is not always the result of humor. People sometimes laugh because they are nervous or angry and do not want to express these emotions. In other cases, people laugh because they think it is the thing to do, such as when someone tells a joke they do not understand. Convention says that it is impolite not to laugh, so the person laughs. The person laughs because she does not want the other person to think she is dumb.

Henman (2001) notes that "communication humor" has been associated with personality traits such as "extroversion, lower anxiety, internal locus of control, and field independence" (p. 90). There is a positive relationship between humor and the ability to communicate emotion or meaning. Those who can use humor effectively present a positive impression.

The importance of humor in social interactions begins in childhood. A study by Sobstad (cited in Fuhr, 2002) found that children who had no humor were likely to play alone. Humor seems to be an important element in social acceptance for status within a group of peers. Other studies have demonstrated that boys who have the highest status among their peers were likely to be the most frequent users of jocular phrases, jokes, and remarks with implicit sexual references (Fuhr, 2002).

Humor and shared laughter can add to feelings of togetherness, warmth, friendliness, and closeness (Astedt-Kurki & Isola, 2001). Humor and laughter can convey a sense of connection between individuals. Social humor may aid in the establishment and development of relationships (Conkell, Imwold, & Ratliffe, 1999). Humor that connects one person to another can help diffuse a stressful

situation. Humor used for stress reduction can be seen in the healthcare setting. For example, when a nurse offers a preoperative patient a hospital gown and says, "Please put on our Paris original." The joking attitude can help ease some of the patient's anxiety.

Provine (2000a) discovered that laughter occurred 30 times more frequently in social situations than solitary situations. This observation was obtained by watching university students' interactions with instructors and with other students. Many of the statements that resulted in laughter were not jokes, but simple statements between individuals, such as "You don't have to drink; just buy us drinks!" Laughter is a signal we send to others. The response of laughter to something mildly humorous seems to disappear when we do not have an audience.

Humor can be used as an interpersonal means of providing comfort. Frecknall (1994) found that the participants in his study felt that humor provided a closeness with others. In a qualitative study by Beck (1997), one theme that emerged was that humor provided an effective therapeutic communication technique that helped to decrease patient anxiety. In a study by Bippus (2000) on humor usage in comforting, all participants were able to recall an interaction in which a friend's use of humor provided an element of comfort during a stressful situation. Humor appears to flow between those who are close, providing an element of release and comfort in times of distress. What happens when the comforter is a stranger, such as in the healthcare setting?

Care providers often attempt to find ways of comforting others (Bippus, 2000). Robinson (1991) notes that humor that "quickly provides a sense of familiarity, does not offend, and is easily facilitated" (p. 51) helps to build a trusting relationship between healthcare providers and patients. Lippert (2001) discovered that humor was an essential part of the relationship between nurses and long-term care residents. Joking tends to strengthen bonds between patients and healthcare providers. An example of this occurred during admission of a same-day surgery patient. The patient had been a regular at the hospital prior to the admission nurse's experience with him. He was an obese man with a reputation for being "obnoxious and difficult." The nurse entered the patient's room with the hospital gown and made a comment about putting on the "Paris original." The patient chuckled and made a humorous comment in response about the gown not covering anything. This interchange established a comfortable relationship between the patient and nurse. As a result, the patient cooperated with the preoperative procedure and was able to share with the nurse his concerns about having surgery.

Gender and Social Hierarchy

An interesting question exists about the differences between the use of humor and humor appreciation between men and women. Is there really a difference? Research does not support a difference in the effects of humor on coping (Abel, 1998). However, response to humor and humor preferences do appear to have some gender-related differences (Provine, 2000b, Robinson & Smith-Lovin, 2001).

A study by Robinson and Smith-Lovin (2001) reports that men tell more jokes than women do. Women joke more with each other when men are not present. Men use humor as a hierarchy-building method. This study indicates that, during group meetings, group members with higher status use more humor and get more laughs than those with lower status. This response seems to support the superiority theory of humor.

Provine (2000b) noticed that women laughed about 126% more than men. Men tended to be the producers of humor. Looking at personal advertisements, Provine noticed that women tended to look for partners with a sense of humor, whereas men were more likely to offer humor. One conclusion

Provine (2000b) made by reviewing his study results and studies of others is that the laughter of women, rather than of men, is the critical index of a healthy relationship.

According to Berk (2002), the following differences exist between men's and women's appreciation of humor:

Men

- Men tend to prefer humor that includes sick, sexual, hostile, cruel, aggressive, disparaging comments and slapstick comedy.

- Watching the Three Stooges beating each other will appeal to more men than women.

- Men prefer humor about bodily functions more than women.

- Men use jokes as a way of holding center stage in a group situation.

Women

- Generally, women prefer noninsulting, nonoffensive types of humor.

- Women are less likely to laugh when someone is hurt or embarrassed.

- Women are often sensitive to any form of humor that is demeaning to their gender.

- Although men make more jokes, women tend to laugh more. This trend may be because women tend to be less inhibited about displaying emotion than men.

- A study of college women indicated that they enjoyed sexual and hostile humor when men were the victims, but not when the victim was female.

- When in a group situation, especially one that includes men, women are less likely to tell jokes than men are.

- If a woman shares jokes in a group they are likely to make warm, witty observations.

- Although some women are very good at telling stories or anecdotes in a humorous way, there are fewer women than men who demonstrate this ability.

Humor and Intimate Relationships

From personal experience most people are aware that humor is an integral part of a close relationship. As noted by Bazzini, Stack, Martincin, and Davis (2006), "One of the most pleasant consequences of spending time with a romantic partner is the opportunity to share humor and subsequently laugh together" (p. 25). Bazzini et al. note that there is little research on maintenance of relationships and humor. In reviewing the literature on humor or laughter and relationships, Bazzini et al. found that couples with lasting, close marital relationships noted that one of the top three reasons for the success of their marriage was the ability to laugh together frequently. The ability to use positive affect, predominately humor and affection, that is demonstrated during conflict situations is a good indicator of the future positive health of a relationship (cited in Driver & Gottman, 2004).

Rabbi Sheldon Moss (2004) used the term "bonding humor" to denote the type of humor that is funny within a relationship that also serves or strengthens relationships and supports bonding between the individuals. Citing from a number of different studies, Moss concluded that humor works as a connection between people, a way for individuals to effectively handle conflicts in a relationship, and to help move a problem into a solution. Humor in relationships can be maladaptive if it is used to avoid discussing issues that get in the way of intimacy; however, it can be adaptive when it becomes part of intimate play.

While interviewing four successfully married couples about humor's role in their marriages as background for developing a humor intervention to teach couples how to effectively use humor as a method of enhancing relationships, Moss learned about bonding through humor as couples shared their experiences. The following are the important psychosocial aspects of this investigation.

"All eight individuals reported peak experiences of emotional openness and physical closeness during poignant episodes of mutually reinforcing laughter" (p. 62). That laughter not only promoted bonding, but the memories of those experiences were seen as the best laughs of a lifetime together. The times of peak laughter seemed to be at times of chaos for the couple and the laughter brought relaxation. The shared laughter seemed to increase closeness and allowed the couple to cope with what could not be controlled.

The laughter between the couples was rarely about canned jokes. It was often about simple situations that required few words to appreciate. Some of the laughter seemed to be about a shared perception of incongruity that was usually unexpected and sometimes it was something that might be socially unacceptable. Moss offers one example of this incongruity experience.

One couple remembered sitting in a dark movie theater when the husband wanted a piece of candy from his wife to soothe his dry throat. She reached into her bag and gave him what she thought was a plastic-covered candy. He had trouble opening it and finally tore it with his teeth. The man put it in his mouth only to find a string hanging out of it. When his wife looked over and saw him with her tampon in his mouth, they both laughed so hard they could not stop, and everyone wanted to kick them out of the movie.

HUMOR AS A COPING STRATEGY AND STRESS RELIEVER

The crisis of today is the joke of tomorrow.
– H.G. Wells

Stress is commonly the result of "stinkin' thinkin." Much of the stress people feel comes from the way they perceive events. When viewing the following, what do you see?

Opportunityisnowhere

Do you see "Opportunity is nowhere" Or do you see "Opportunity is now here" How do you perceive the message?

We all perceive that there is stress in our lives. Of course, without some element of stress, we would stop functioning because stress keeps us breathing and our heart beating. It is the excess stress that becomes the problem. It is the sense of carrying the world on our shoulders that leads to our need to find effective methods of releasing that stress.

The meaning an individual places on a situation influences how the person feels about the situation. If a person tells himself or herself that a certain event is terrible, he or she will react to that stressor in a negative manner. A person's reaction to stress

Note. From MentalHealthHumor.com. Used with permission from Chato B. Stewart.

may manifest itself physically, psychologically, socially, and even spiritually. Emotionally, stress can manifest as moodiness, inability to concentrate, irritability, changes in eating or sleeping patterns, crying, decreased libido, worrying, mood swings, frustration, nervousness, and depression. Individuals may also display a negative attitude, lack of creativity, lethargy, low productivity, confusion, boredom, or forgetfulness (Buxman, 1998). They may isolate themselves from others or feel a sense of loneliness. Preoccupation with stressful events can lead to negative mood swings, lashing out at others, nagging, or distancing oneself from and not talking to others.

Lefcourt and Martin (1986) believe that humor and laughter are "an important mechanism for coping with many of the psychological stressors that humans encounter in their daily lives" (p. 1). It is believed that humor helps to decrease the sense of stress by producing a cognitive shift or by helping to restructure how a person views a situation (Abel, 1998). In other words, humor provides a different perspective on stressful situations. It gives people a sense of control over their environments and offers a sense of self-protection (Wooten, 1996). Humor helps people view stressful situations in more positive and challenging ways by helping to refocus attention on less-negative aspects of the situation (Kuiper, Martin, & Olinger, 1993). One of the themes from Frecknall's (1994) qualitative study was that "humor provides significant and often unexpected release from stress" (p. 17).

How negative life events impact individuals depends on such variables as coping strategies and hardiness (Porterfield, 1987). Wooten (1996) refers to the issue of internal versus external locus of control. Individuals with external loci of control believe that things happen to them that are beyond their control. Those who have internal loci of control believe they have some control over what happens to them; these people are more likely to take control of their own health care. Wooten's (1996) study indicated that individuals who were encouraged to use humor developed a sense of control in their lives. This sense of control made individuals more willing to follow recommended health interventions. Wooten (1997) mentioned that her observations led her to believe that patients with good senses of humor or playful spirits have a resilience and strength that helps them deal with the difficult and frightening moments of illness.

In 2007, Petzall and Olsson shared a humor intervention study done in Sweden with two groups of older adults. One group lived at home and the other group lived in a sheltered accommodation. Each group of volunteers older than age 60 was involved in a humor circle. They were assigned to bring in humorous true life stories to share. Each group took the Psychological General Well-Being questionnaire before and after the intervention. The result of this experiment was that the sense of well-being for those who lived at home did not rise significantly, while that of those living in the sheltered accommodation facility did. The authors felt that the difference was that those living at home had plenty of opportunity to interact with others, whereas those living in a sheltered environment had to work a little harder to seek out others for suggestions for stories, thereby increasing their interaction with others. Apparently this was a positive experience for both groups because two humor circles were formed in the sheltered accommodation because others wanted to be involved. The senior center that recruited the at-home population for the study also started two humor circles.

In the above study, neither group had improvement in physical health, but for the sheltered group the sense of being healthy improved. The sheltered group also demonstrated decreased feelings of depression and increased vitality. In order to bring humorous stories to the humor circle, individuals interacted with others. Those living in the sheltered accommodation had to seek the assistance of other residents and staff as well as family, thereby increasing their social connections. This was not the case for those living at home because they were active in the community. Because humor and laughter usually occur in social situations, it is easy to understand how this type of intervention would improve the sense of well-being for those whose social circle had become limited.

Martin and Lefcourt (1983) designed three quantitative studies using different measures of sense of humor and its effect on moderating the impact of stressful events. All three studies provided initial evidence that humor played a role in buffering stress. The researchers also found an inverse relationship between humor production and life stressors and between humor production and negative mood. Plus, subjects who reported high stress levels also reported producing and using more humor.

The first study used three different humor assessment tools, each of which measured somewhat different aspects of the complex sense of humor constructs. The researchers used the Life Events of College Students and Profile of Mood States questionnaires to determine level of stress and feelings of tension, depression, anger, fatigue, and confusion. This study indicated that individuals who tend to smile and laugh in a wide variety of situations place a high value on the use of humor, and those who state they use humor as a means of coping with stressful events have less pronounced mood disturbance from the effects of stress. The second study, which used a self-report measure of sense of humor, also indicated that humor had a stress-buffering effect. The same result was evident in the third study, in which participants were instructed to make up humorous statements for a silent film and then complete a questionnaire. This study indicated that neither the ability to accurately perceive humorous stimuli in one's environment nor reports of humor appreciation were significant for humor to decrease or moderate the effect of stress. However, those who placed a high value on humor for handling difficult situations and were able to produce humorous stories demonstrated significantly lower levels of mood disturbances.

Since the 1983 study by Martin and Lefcourt, other quantitative studies on the use of humor have demonstrated decreases in anxiety and interruption in the cycle of stress (Moran, 1996, Pasquali, 1990). A study looking at nursing strategies that activate hopefulness in adolescents diagnosed with oncologic illness revealed that nurses who employed a light-hearted and playful attitude promoted feelings of hopefulness (Hunt, 1993). This study supports the positive influence humor has on feelings of hopefulness. Bellert (1989) reminds us that shared humor and laughter can enhance communication. "[Humor and laughter] allow the patient to consider alternative ways of looking at life, of exploring new coping skills, and of gaining control over health" (Bellert, 1989, p. 69). Bokun (1986) states that humor used as therapy when dealing with cancer patients offers nothing to lose but worries.

Kuiper, Martin, and Olinger (1993) performed a study looking at humor and cognitive appraisal of potentially stressful events using academic examinations. The study confirmed the theories that those with higher humor scores would be able to use humor effectively to distance themselves from stressful life events. Individuals who scored as high humor users were found to deal with stressful situations in a more direct fashion. The study also revealed that people with high humor scores tended to be less vulnerable to threats to their self-esteem than those with lower humor scores.

A study by Labott and Martin (1987) on the moderating effects of emotional weeping and humor on negative life events revealed that, in all but the male group who reported weeping frequently, those who used humor found that it helped to decrease the intensity of a negative experience. Martin and Lefcourt (1983) reported that, as negative life events increase, people using humor to cope report less mood disturbances than individuals who are less likely to use humor. Labott, Ahleman,

Wolever, and Martin (1990) also discovered that using humor to cope was associated with more positive moods.

Two studies by Lefcourt, Davidson, Shepherd, Phillips, Prakachin, and Mills (1995) looked at ways in which humor could account for the stress-moderating effects found in other humor studies. The researchers looked at perspective-taking humor. Perspective-taking humor is defined as "a readiness to assume a remote and comic vision of ourselves" (Lefcourt et al., 1995, p. 387). Most of the subjects in these studies reported dysphoria after taking part in stress-producing, death-related activities. Those individuals who rated high in perspective-taking humor showed little change in affect. The studies also revealed that individuals who were able to understand and enjoy the cartoons used in the studies had positive emotional effects. Lefcourt and colleagues (1995) concluded that people who can envision their lives from a remote perspective may be better able to think about catastrophic events without becoming excessively distressed. This study was conducted using humor as a means of coping with stressful events, indicating that humor may offer a means of reframing how we see ourselves in situations that are related to death.

It has been argued that laughter and crying are both cathartics – measures that can be used to release tension (Goodheart, 1994). Labott and Martin (1987) looked at the effects of crying and humor on stress modification. Crying did not prove to be a buffer against life stress in the college students who participated. Humor, on the other hand, did prove to buffer life stress in all categories except males categorized by high crying.

A study by Makinen, Suominen, and Lauri (2000) investigated the mechanisms that help adult asthma patients cope with their disease. They found that social support played a significant part in patients' ability to fight a sense of powerlessness. Ninety-one percent said that humor helped them cope with psychological self-care, whereas 80% said that positive thinking helped. On the humor scale, 49 people said they totally agreed that humor helped, 42 said they agreed that it helped, 9 were not sure, and only 1 said humor did not help. Of all the parameters this study researched regarding psychological self-care (positive thinking, finding time for self, exercise, actively pushing aside negative thinking, crying, and humor) the only parameter that no one checked as "totally disagree" was humor.

Concerns about coping strategies used by caregivers of pediatric patients led Wade, Borawski, Taylor, Drotar, Yeates, and Stancin (2001) to investigate the types of coping mechanisms used by parents of children who experienced traumatic brain injury (TBI) and children with orthopedic injuries. One of the strategies investigated was the use of humor. This study was the first to look at specific outcomes of caregiver and family coping during the initial year following pediatric injury. It was also the first to look at differences in the severity of injury, coping strategies, and caregiver and family outcomes. The study sample included 109 children with moderate-to-severe TBI and 80 children with orthopedic injuries that had no central nervous system insult. The parent most likely to take part in the study was the mother.

Overall, emotion-focused coping strategies (of which humor was one of the mechanisms) were associated with better caregiver and family outcomes, whereas denial and disengagement were associated with more negative outcomes (Wade et al., 2001). The relationship between coping and caregiver response varied depending on the severity of the injury. This indicates that certain coping strategies may be influenced by the nature of the stressor. Of the coping mechanisms investigated, humor use reduced caregiver distress from 6 to 12 months after TBI, but it did not have the same effect following orthopedic injuries. This finding could be because orthopedic injuries are self-limiting, and TBI requires many different adjustments and

remains a prevailing experience in the life of the child and family. It is possible that coming to terms with the multiple problems, or even joking about them, may let the caregiver cope more effectively with sequelae of the injury.

A news article in *USA Today* by Marilyn Elias (2003) discusses the possibility that happy people live longer than unhappy people. Elias quotes a study that reported that happy adults with heart disease are 20% more likely than unhappy adults with heart disease to live another 11 years. The reason for this difference in survival is not clear; however, researchers hypothesize that positive emotions do not trigger stress hormones which can make blood platelets thicker and thicken the blood.

Ongoing research by the Baltimore Longitudinal Study of Aging indicates that cheerful people complain less about chest pain. Also, unhappy people are more likely to isolate themselves, not take their medications as prescribed, eat less healthy and are less likely to exercise than cheerful people. In other words, people who can find things to be joyful about are more likely to live fuller, happier, and longer lives. Humor is one way to put a new perspective on negative events in life, and it helps maintain a sense of happiness.

Humor can also be used to help people distance themselves from stressful situations. For example, Nazi prisoners used humor as a survival mechanism (Frankl, 1963; Henman, 2001). Henman's (2001) study of prisoners of the Vietnam war indicates the importance of humor as a stress-reduction method as well as a survival mechanism. In an online article about humor during the war with Iraq, Dr. Paul Wong (2003) states, "Humor also allows one to move from rigidity to openness, from despair to hope, and from fear to the celebration of life. With humor and laughter, we not only cope better, but also become healthier and happier."

DEATH, BEREAVEMENT, AND HUMOR

Bereavement is a painful process for mourners. Mourning saps energy and causes feelings of depression and possibly fear. Humor can offer some relief to the pain of grief and can decrease depression and improve energy levels. For some, the best way to understand the benefits of laughter is through stories of those who have used humor to cope. Herth (1995) tells one such story about a funeral she attended for a 68-year-old gentleman she had cared for through a hospice program:

This particular gentleman had a great sense of humor and had always been the "life of a party." Prior to entering the sanctuary of the church, the family, close friends, and myself were secluded in a room just off to the side. The silence in the room was deafening. The minister asked if anyone wanted to ask or say anything before we went into the church. Remembering his joy for living, I asked if anyone could think of specific times they had spent with him that brought a sense of delight and joy to the heart that we could share before entering the sanctuary. One of the family members shared a humorous, joyful time they had together, and immediately other members shared similar experiences. The family and friends recognized that this gentleman would want his funeral to be a celebration of his life and his joy for living…Several weeks later, several family members and friends told me how much it had meant to share the joyous moments at the funeral, and how important this was to them as they were working through the grieving process (pp. 222-223).

Humor is one way members of bereavement groups can connect with one another and share their respective grief. During the seventh meeting of an 8-week bereavement group, a female member shared that friends of hers were taking her to a club that had male strippers. They had decided it was time for her to "let go and cut up" a little. Another member of the group, an elderly gentleman who had lost his wife of 62 years, perked up as she was talking. Someone started teasing her about putting money in the dancer's G-string. Suddenly, this gentleman, who was usually very quiet, said, "Would you put money in my G-string if I danced for you?" Everyone started to laugh. The next week, at the final meeting, which consisted of a pizza dinner, the participants were still laughing and teasing both of them about the week before. The gentleman who had been so depressed and quiet was laughing and participating in the fun. The gentleman's response was a good indication of the beginning of a healing process. It was wonderful to see the difference a little bit of humor made in the lives of the woman and the older gentleman as well as the other participants.

CASE STUDY

*M*rs. *Green, a 64-year-old retired sales clerk, has been admitted to a rehabilitation unit following an above-the-knee amputation of her right leg. Her physician has switched her from oral antidiabetic agents to insulin only. She also has a history of mild chronic obstructive pulmonary disease. Her family describes her as an "easygoing, cheerful, social" person. Since Mrs. Green has been on the unit, she refuses to leave her room except to go to physical therapy. When not doing her exercises she lies in bed facing the wall with her covers pulled up to her chin. She laughingly refers to her room as her "cave."*

Questions

1. Is her laughter a positive coping mechanism? Explain.

2. What assessments are important when planning humor interventions with her?

3. What behavior changes would indicate that the humor interventions are effective?

Discussion

Mrs. Green's comment about her room being her cave is a clue that she is depressed and her laughter is due to something other than amusement. This type of laughter is not an effective coping mechanism because it is not relieving her depression. As far as intervention goes, it would be best for the healthcare provider to explore what the underlying issue is before making an attempt to plan a humor intervention. Was she grieving the loss of her leg? Is she grieving life as she knew it and making assumptions about what life is going to be like without her leg? What self-image issues are involved with the surgery? After the underlying issues are dealt with, the care provider can begin to explore Mrs. Green's former coping mechanisms and introduce the aspect of humor. As Mrs. Green's depression begins to lift, finding ways to add gentle humor by paying attention to comments, encouraging the family to start joking with her, and being sensitive to those comments she finds amusing would be helpful. Offering her humorous stories to read, being aware of when she watches sitcoms and talking about them, and maybe even doing something humorous about her "cave" are interventions that might be helpful. When Mrs. Green presents as the "easygoing, cheerful, social" person the family remembers, the care provider can assess that the interventions have been successful.

SUMMARY

The psychosocial aspects of humor are important elements in coping with life stress and relationship formation. Humor helps people connect with one another. It is a great communicator. It also helps put life events into perspective. Studies by Frecknall (1994) and Beck (1997) demonstrate the use of humor as a form of connection between people. The participants in Bippus's (2000) study claimed that humor was comforting during stressful situations. Lippert's (2001) study demonstrates that humor is essential to the relationships that develop between nurses and long-term care residents. These studies, and others, indicate the importance of using humor to build relationships.

There are differences between men and women's use of humor. Knowledge of these differences is helpful in understanding how differences can enhance or detract from a relationship. It also helps to understand how one type of humor might result in a mirth response leading to relaxation in men and tension in women, or visa versa.

Positive relationships are an important part of patient care. Whether the patient is dealing with a non-terminal illness, or at the last stages of the life process, humor offers an outlet for stress and builds relationships between the healthcare provider and the patient. Klein (1998) says that "humor helps us keep our balance when life throws us a curve ball" (p. 4). Using humor in the healthcare setting may help patients "keep their balance."

EXAM QUESTIONS

CHAPTER 6
Questions 44-51

Note: Choose the one option that BEST answers each question.

44. Humor is important in social situations because it

   a. can help hide a person's fears.

   b. helps a person become more popular.

   c. helps a person breathe better when stress occurs.

   d. improves communication by dissolving barriers.

45. When nurses use humor judiciously with patients it

   a. helps increase rapport between the nurse and patient.

   b. lets the patient know that the nurse is in charge.

   c. tells the patient that everything will be all right.

   d. increases the game of pretend so patients feel less stress.

46. Using humor in serious situations

   a. is always appropriate in any situation.

   b. is never appropriate in any situation.

   c. might be helpful if used carefully.

   d. is always hurtful to the person involved in the situation.

47. A patient says to his nurse, "The doctor says my disease is terminal. I guess I better cash in my bonds," and starts to laugh. The best action by the healthcare provider is to

   a. laugh with the patient and then leave.

   b. ask an open-ended question to assess level of distress.

   c. ask the patient if he would like to speak to a social worker.

   d. ask the patient if he would like something from the humor cart.

48. When examining gender and social hierarchy in humor, studies have shown

   a. members of a group with higher status use more humor and get more laughs.

   b. members of a group with lower status tell more jokes.

   c. women tell more jokes than men.

   d. men laugh at jokes more than women.

49. One positive effect of using humor in intimate relationships during times of stress is that

   a. people who laugh together always stay together.

   b. it prevents others from disturbing the relationship.

   c. it improves the ability to tell jokes.

   d. it helps strengthen the relationship and support interpersonal coping.

50. One of the most significant advantages to the use of humor in stressful situations is that it

    a. resolves the problem.

    b. prevents mood swings.

    c. can change a person's perspective.

    d. can lead to laughter.

51. The use of humor in a bereavement group

    a. helps members connect/share their grief.

    b. prevents people from coping with a death.

    c. avoids telling stories of the deceased.

    d. increases anxiety about death.

CHAPTER 7

THE PHYSIOLOGICAL EFFECTS OF HUMOR

Laughter is the sensation of feeling good all over and showing it principally in one place.

– Josh Billings

CHAPTER OBJECTIVE

After completing this chapter, the reader will be able to describe how humor can affect the immune system, physiological health, and pain management.

LEARNING OBJECTIVES

After studying this chapter, the reader will be able to

1. articulate the body's normal response to stress.

2. identify the immunological changes caused by humor.

3. describe how humor may affect cardiac and respiratory well-being.

4. describe the use of humor as an adjunct therapy in pain management.

INTRODUCTION

It is known that humor has a physiological effect on the human body. The interest in how humor and laughter affect the body has led to a relatively new area of study termed gelotology. This chapter will look at the physiological changes that occur with mirth and laughter according to studies and scientific theories. As the reader ponders the reported results, it is important to remember that many of the studies have small participant sizes. There is also a short discussion on psychoneuroimmunology, the study of how the mind and body are interconnected.

PHYSIOLOGICAL STRESS REACTION

Stressful life events cause the autonomic nervous system to prepare for "fight or flight." The body's physiological stress reaction is diagramed in Figure 7-1.

When a person experiences acute physical or emotional stress, the adrenal gland increases its secretion of cortisol. Increased heart rate and blood pressure enhance blood flow to the skeletal muscles, enabling the person to flee the situation. The cortisol increase also increases appetite. As a result, fat breaks down to provide energy to the muscles. Production of dehydroepiandrosterone (DHEA), a steroid that helps buffer the body against the effects of excess cortisol, also increases. This buffer works as a protective mechanism during times of acute stress.

When a person perceives a threat, real or imagined, the body activates the general adaptation syndrome (GAS). During the alarm reaction of the GAS, the hypothalamus-pituitary-adrenal (HPA)

FIGURE 7-1: PHYSIOLOGICAL STRESS REACTION

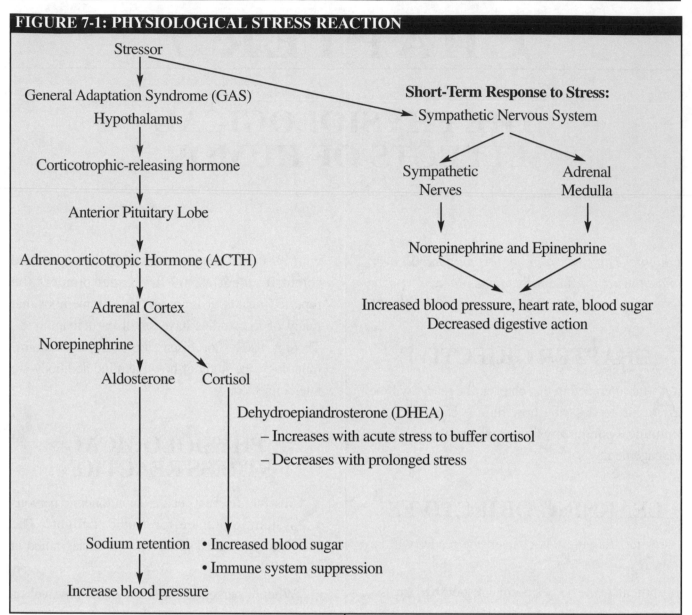

axis is activated. The anterior pituitary gland releases adrenocorticotropic hormone (ACTH) which, in turn, increases the secretion of cortisol from the adrenal gland into the systemic circulation. A complex feedback mechanism within the immune and endocrine systems works to further regulate HPA function, preventing excessive secretion of cortisol and ACTH. Epinephrine and norepinephrine are released due to stimulation of the adrenal medulla. The heart rate is raised and the blood vessels constrict.

Also known as the *stress response,* fight-or-flight syndrome worked well when humans were hunters and gatherers. It allowed the body to quickly change from quiet waiting to a rapid physical response. However, emotional stress causes overstimulation of the HPA axis and can lead to physiological changes that have detrimental effects on the body. With long periods of stress, DHEA levels fall, leaving high cortisol levels unchecked. High levels of cortisol can create immunosuppression, leaving the body more susceptible to infection and disease.

When an individual experiences a stressful life event, his or her muscles become tense. The person may develop a headache, clench the jaw, grind the teeth, or experience tightness in the neck, shoulder, and back muscles. The digestive system is affected and loss of appetite, abdominal discomfort, nausea, vomiting, diarrhea, and irritable bowel syndrome may occur. Tension can also lead to heart attacks. Ford-Martin (2001) notes that 80% to 90% of all diseases are believed to be stress related.

Risk factors for stress-related illnesses include a mix of personal, interpersonal, and social variables. These factors can include lack or loss of social support or an actual or perceived loss of control over one's physical environment. A stress response can occur with negative life events, such as the death of a loved one or loss of a job. It can also occur with life events that are viewed as positive, such as getting married, attending finishing school, becoming a parent, or entering into retirement. It has also been found that people who are dependent on others, such as children or the elderly, and those who are socially disadvantaged because of race, gender, educational level, or similar factors are at great risk for developing stress-related diseases (Ford-Martin, 2001).

"You're under too much stress. Have you considered leaving your librarian job?"

Note. From DansCartoons.com. Used with permission.

IMMUNE RESPONSE TO HUMOR

Many research studies have been conducted on the immunological effects of humor. Some researchers, however, are concerned with the methodology used (Martin, 2001). This research has been criticized for inadequate sample sizes and other methodological weaknesses. Although the scientific evidence is inadequate to state with certainty that response to humor can cause changes in the immune system, these studies do provide clues as to how humor can affect the immune system and can be used to design further research studies with stronger statistical power. From a health care perspective, it is important to ask, "Is it worth trying something fun that might help boost immune function?"

A quick review of immune system properties that may be affected by humor can help you to understand how humor can be used in health care (see Table 7-1). Research indicates that humor increases the immunoglobulin IgA. Studies also indicate that IgG, IgM, killer T cells, and natural killer (NK) cells increase with laughter (Berk et al., 1989; Berk, Felten, Tan, Bittman, & Westengard, 2001). Sedimentation rate and the amount of cortisol in blood reportedly decrease as a result of laughter. All of these effects have potential benefits for patients.

One of the best-known studies that examined the immunological effects of humor and laughter was conducted by Berk and associates in 1989 and was replicated in 1993. Although there are some questions about methodology regarding control groups (Martin, 2001), these studies indicate that humor has some definite immunological benefits. The following points summarize the effects of humor on the immune system according to the studies of Berk and associates:

- IgG increases with hearty laughter and remains elevated for 24 hours.

TABLE 7-1: IMMUNE SYSTEM PROPERTIES AND THEIR FUNCTIONS

Property	Function
Immunoglobulins	Respond to antigen release, such as bacteria and viruses.
IgG	Major immunoglobulin in blood. Coats microorganisms and speeds their uptake by cells in the immune system. Responsible for producing long-term immunity.
IgA	Found in saliva, tears, secretions of gastrointestinal and respiratory tracts and guard entrances to the body to protect against colds and flu.
IgM	Found in bloodstream. First antibody to arrive during hormonal response. Kills bacteria.
Complement 3	Helps antibodies penetrate and destroy defective or infective cells.
T cells	Help organize immune system responses.
Helper T	Mobilize many immune cells, especially B and T cells.
Killer T cells	Fight off invading organisms, especially viruses and cells transformed by cancer.
Suppressor T cells	Help stop T cell reaction when T cells are no longer needed.
Phagocytes	White blood cells that engulf and digest foreign invaders.
B cells	Produced by the bone marrow. Generate antibodies to fight potentially harmful microorganisms.
Natural killer (NK) cells	Attack viruses and tumor cells.
Cytokines	Small proteins that are released from cells. Act as messengers to other cells. Actively involved in the immune response.
Gamma interferon	Specialized hormone-like product. Regulates anticellular activities and turns on mononuclear lymphocytes (white blood cells).

- IgA and IgM also increase, and levels stay elevated into the next day.

- Mirthful laughter increases NK cell activity and increases the actual number of cells.

- Gamma interferon increases twofold as subjects watch a humor video.

Along with changes in the amounts of IgA, IgG, IgM, T cells, and NK cells, cortisol secretion decreased. As cortisol increases in the body, immune defenses decrease. Therefore, a decrease in cortisol should increase the immune system's ability to respond. The level of B cells also increased when subjects watched a comedy video. This result is not surprising because B cells are responsible for the production of immunoglobulins.

Another study of ten students revealed a significant increase in salivary IgA after students viewed a humorous videotape (Groves, 1991). This study on salivary IgA and perceived mood over a number of weeks revealed that IgA concentrations were high on days the subjects perceived they were in a positive mood. On days the individuals perceived themselves to be in a negative mood, the salivary concentrations were lower. Another interesting finding was that IgA levels were "directly related to the subjects' perceptions of their use of humor as a coping device" (Groves, 1991, p. 52). Those who viewed themselves as using humor for coping did not have as high an increase in IgA after viewing the humorous film as those who did not use humor as a coping device. Another study noted that people who stated they used humor to cope had higher baseline levels of IgA, even though watching a laughter film had no effect on levels of immunoglobulins (Martin, 2001).

In a series of studies by Berk and colleagues (2001), blood samples collected before and after humor interventions showed that laughter had a positive immunologic effect (see Table 7-2).

People who had high scores on the Humor Response Scale (HRS) and mirthful laughter were found to have increased levels of NK cell activity. The ability to increase NK cell activity through the use of humor may have clinical significance in the treatment of viral disease and cancer (Bennett, Zeller, Rosenberg, & McCann, 2003).

OTHER PHYSIOLOGICAL EFFECTS OF HUMOR

Think about what happens when someone laughs:

* The person takes in big breaths of air, and then blows them out.

* The stomach moves and perhaps the person's whole body begins to move.

* If the person laughs very hard, his or her face may turn red.

All of this activity that occurs with laughter may have some important physiological benefits. For example, a postoperative patient who laughs at the antics of a hospital clown laughs, coughs, and then laughs again at the clown's antics. The coughing helps clear the lungs, and the laughter is much more fun than using an incentive spirometer.

In an interview with Patty Wooten (1994), Dr. Fry stated that laughter "disturbed the usual pattern of respiration, increased the minute volume, and created a forceful exhalation which could mobilize secretions." Laughter is believed to work on the respiratory system by triggering a bellows action on the thoracic cavity. Laughter did not, however, increase oxygen saturation. Fry also noted that laughter aids ventilation and the cleansing of mucus from the lungs. This finding might help those with certain chronic respiratory conditions. Plus, large muscle masses are activated during laughter, which creates a total body response that may be useful in providing conditioning exercises for bed-ridden or wheelchair-bound patients.

Consider the dissection of laughter by Kuhn (2003). He talks about 15 stages of laughter (see Table 7-3). While reading about each stage, think about what part of the body is being exercised.

Berk (2002) notes that 15 facial muscles are used with a hearty guffaw, and the skeletal muscles contract. Laughter creates a total body response. Berk (2002) also mentions that a belly laugh exercises the chest and abdominal muscles, improving their tone. This exercise can be important for wheelchair-bound or bed-ridden patients. Use of the abdominal muscles during hearty laughter can also affect the gastrointestinal system and may improve digestion. During laughter, normal cyclic breathing is disrupted, ventilation increases, mucus plugs may

TABLE 7-2: EFFECTS OF HUMOR AND LAUGHTER ON IMMUNE SYSTEM	
Immune System Component	**Effects**
Natural killer cells (NK)	Increase activity, especially in experimental subjects
IgG, IgA, IgM	Increases after 30 minutes, remains elevated 90 minutes and 12 hours after intervention
Complement 3	Significant increase 90 minutes after intervention
T cells	Increase activity during intervention and remain for at least 90 minutes
B cells	Increase significantly at 90 minutes and remain up to 12 hours
Helper T cells	Increase during intervention and remain elevated up to 12 hours
Cytokine gamma interferon	Significant increase at 90 minutes and remains elevated up to 12 hours
Total leukocytes	Increases during and 90 minutes after intervention

TABLE 7-3: 15 STAGES OF LAUGHTER

1. **Smirk:** This is the often fleeting, slight upturning of the corners of the mouth and a gentle hint of openness in the eyes. It is completely voluntary and controlled. It is commonly hard to detect.

2. **Smile:** This is usually voluntary, silent, controlled, and easily noticed. The corners of the mouth turn upward and the eyes sparkle.

3. **Grin:** This is also silent and controlled but uses more facial muscles. The corners of the mouth are stretched upward, and the cheeks are involved.

4. **Snicker:** This involves the first emergence of sound accompanied by facial movement. It is accompanied by sounds caused by bursts of air released from the nose.

5. **Giggle:** This usually tickles us inside and is expressed outwardly in sound.It involves a series of rapid, often high-pitched sounds. The sound of giggling can be amusing. The attempt to suppress it tends to increase its strength.

6. **Chuckle:** This involves the chest muscles, and the sound has a deeper pitch. The sound is similar "to a dog whose bark is caught in his throat" (Kuhn, 2003, p. 36). The sound seems to come from the back of the throat.

7. **Chortle:** This response originates deeper in the chest and involves the torso muscles. It usually provokes laughter in others.

8. **Laugh:** By the time the process reaches the laugh, it is irreversible. The laugh involves facial and thoracic muscles as well as the abdomen and extremities. Sounds of barking or snorting may occur.

9. **Cackle:** At this point, the process is involuntary. The pitch of the sound is higher, the body begins to rock, the spine extends and flexes, and the head becomes upturned. Kuhn (2003) refers to this sound as "a laugh on pep pills."

10. **Guffaw:** At this stage, the whole body responds. Feet stomp, arms wave, and the person may slap his or her thighs. The torso rocks and the sound that emerges is deep and loud. "It is incompatible with a full bladder" (Kuhn, 2003, pg. 37).

11. **Howl:** The body becomes more animated as the volume and pitch rise higher and higher.

12. **Shriek:** The intensity increases. There is a sense of vulnerability and helplessness.

13. **Roar:** By this time, the audience is also roaring. Individuality is lost.

14. **Convulse:** The body is completely out of control in a fit of laughter that resembles a seizure. Extremities flail aimlessly. The person loses balance, starts gasping for breath, and collapses or falls off the chair.

15. **Die laughing:** This is a brief, physically intense experience in which there is an instant of total helplessness. It is a transcendent experience. The person is totally powerless, defenseless, and incapable of purposeful movement. After the experience, it is as if the person is reborn.

"You have nothing left…Like a newborn infant, you may be physically weak and lack coordination. All of your senses may be refreshed and sharpened. And, in some instances, you may need a change of underwear" (Kuhn, 2003, p. 38).

(Kuhn, 2003)

clear, and residual air exchange is accelerated. Increased pulmonary ventilation results in blowing off excess carbon dioxide and water vapor that builds up in residual air. Fry contends that laughter allows more oxygen availability for red blood cell uptake in addition to decreasing moisture, thereby preventing pulmonary bacterial growth (Berk, 2002).

Studies looking at the effects of humor on patients with chronic obstructive pulmonary disease

(COPD) indicated an increased functional residual capacity (FRC) secondary to increased air trapping. This situation was most noticeable in patients with less severe pulmonary disease. Additionally, COPD patients with humorous coping styles were found to have less depression and anxiety, fewer infections, and enhanced quality of life. Because the act of laughing out loud may cause negative pulmonary function, humor should be used cautiously with COPD patients (Lebowitz, 2002).

If humor affects COPD, what are the effects on patients with allergies? A small study by Maranan (2001) indicates that laughter might be one way of decreasing allergic symptoms in some people.

Dr. Fry decided to investigate the effect of laughter on the body. Dr. Fry believes that venous return is enhanced partly by the milking action of active muscles on the venous system (Wooten, 1994). Laughter initially causes an increase in heart rate, blood pressure, and respiratory rate. It also works the face and stomach muscles and relaxes muscles that are not involved in laughing (Dossey, 1996). Using himself as a subject, Fry found that 1 minute of hearty laughter brought his heart rate up to the same level as 10 minutes of rowing on his home rowing machine. Which would be more enjoyable: hearty laughter or rowing for 10 minutes?

How are patients who experienced a myocardial infarction (MI) affected by humor? Researchers followed two groups of patients for 1 year of cardiac rehabilitation. They found that patients who viewed self-selected humor films had fewer episodes of arrhythmias, lower blood pressure, lower urinary and plasma catecholamines, less need for beta blockers and nitroglycerin, and a lower incidence of recurrent MI than the control group who did not watch humorous material (Tan, Tan, Berk, Lukman, & Lukman, 1997).

According to the University of Maryland Medical Center (2005), a recent study indicates that emotions appear to have an effect on the inner lining of blood vessels, the endothelium. Viewing a movie that provoked laughter had the effect of dilating blood vessels and increasing blood flow. In contrast, viewing movie clips that tended to cause mental stress resulted in a decreased brachial artery flow. The study was unable to determine the source of laughter's benefit. It might be caused by the movement of the diaphragm muscles when a person chuckles or guffaws, or a chemical release triggered by the laughter. Whatever the cause, the researchers believe this study adds to the evidence that there is a connection between laughter and cardiovascular health.

In reviewing the differences between men who used humor and men who were less likely to use humor in their daily lives, it was found that humor users had a lower incidence of cardiac disease (Jancin, 2001). This study indicates that a good sense of humor may be cardioprotective. It is believed that laughter might help keep hearts healthy by "helping to decrease blood vessel inflammation, decreasing the risk of clots, or helping to maintain normal blood pressure levels" (Walsh, n.d., p. 3).

Sahakian and Frishman (2007) note that evidence indicates intense laughter may cause sudden increases in blood pressure that could be dangerous for those at risk of cerebrovascular accidents (CVAs). However, there are no reported cases of CVAs or heart attacks in the literature from intense laughter. It is possible that the contraction of the skeletal muscles occurring from laughter might actually increase venous return via a milking effect, thereby decreasing the risk of venous stasis and blood clots. The difficulty in predicting effects of humor on patients with cardiovascular compromises is that all studies to date have been conducted on healthy patients or have looked at acute effects of humor. More studies need to be conducted in order to scientifically claim that humor is physiologically helpful for those patients with cardiovascular history.

Researchers at the University of Maryland (2005) reported study results that indicated laughter appeared to cause the endothelium, the tissue forming the inner lining of the blood vessels, to dilate or expand. The dilation of the blood vessels would allow an increased blood flow throughout the body. Since the endothelium is the first line in the development of atherosclerosis (hardening of the arteries) this study indicates that laughter might be one way of maintaining a healthy endothelium and decreasing the risk of cardiovascular disease.

An article by Ara Sahakian and William Frishman (2007) summarizes what is known about humor's affect on the cardiovascular system. From the studies it is fair to conclude that changes do occur (Table 7-4). These changes all occurred on healthy adults.

What effect will viewing a comedy show have on the blood sugar of patients with diabetes? An interesting study conducted on 19 patients with type 2 diabetes suggests that a significant suppression of 2-hour postprandial blood glucose (PPBG) level occurred after watching a comedy show (Hayashi et al., 2003). As noted by the authors, negative emotions, such as fear, anxiety, or sorrow, tend to elevate blood glucose levels. The results of this study indicate that laughter has an inhibitory effect on the increase in PPBG. The reason for this effect is not clear, but Hayashi et al. (2003) have two different theories for this phenomenon:

1. the acceleration of glucose used by the muscle motion while laughing and

2. positive emotions, such as laughter, act on the neuroendocrine system and suppress the elevation of blood glucose levels.

Because this is probably the first study conducted on blood glucose and the sample size was small, more studies need to be done.

One word of caution: Some people have experienced negative physiological effects to laughter (Berk et al., 2001). A small number of people experience neurological reactions to laughter. These reactions include seizures and cataleptic and narcoleptic attacks. Following abdominal surgery or pelvic surgery, laughter may be contraindicated because increased abdominal and thoracic pressure can occur (thus the phrase 'bust a gut'). This increase in pressure can also have negative consequences for those with respiratory diseases such as asthma.

HUMOR AND PAIN MANAGEMENT

When you're hungry, sing; when you're hurt, laugh.
– Jewish Proverb

Interest in the effects of laughter on pain control arose after Norman Cousins (1979) shared his experience of using humor to control his pain level during his recovery from ankylosing spondylitis. Cousins found that he could control his pain by reading humorous books and watching Marx Brothers films and Candid Camera productions. He found that 10 minutes of belly laughter left him pain free for about 2 hours.

TABLE 7-4: ACUTE EFFECTS OF LAUGHTER ON THE CARDIOVASCULAR SYSTEM IN HEALTHY ADULTS	
Beta-adrenergic stimulation – affects vasodilation and heart rate – Too much stimulation appears to cause increased blood pressure and feelings of anxiety	Decreased
Venous return	Increased
Brachial artery flow – mediated vasodilation	Increased
Blood oxygen saturation	No change

Modified from Sahakian & Frishman, 2007.

Like humor, pain is a perception. This perception affects people's emotions. If the mind and body are inseparable, then one cannot feel pain physiologically without some emotional effect. It is known that pain is changeable and variable. Different people perceive pain differently depending on past experiences with pain, cultural expectations of pain, the meaning of a situation to that person (some people are incapacitated by pain and others might just find it annoying), and other stressors affecting tension within the body.

The actual physiological process that affects the pain level following laughter is still not known. It is believed that laughter helps by providing a distraction, reducing tension, changing expectations, and possibly increasing production of endogenous endorphins – the body's own morphine (Rosner, 2002). The belief that endorphins are released has not been demonstrated in research studies according to the literature search conducted for this text.

A number of controlled studies used a noxious stimulus during the viewing of humorous material to determine if laughter had any effect on pain levels (Provine, 2000a). The noxious stimulation included a mild electric current applied to participants' forearms, blood pressure cuff inflation, or cold-pressor tasks (such as placing the hands in ice water). The end results of these controlled studies indicated that pain threshold is increased with laughter. There is also speculation that mirthful laughter increases endorphins; however, so far, no definitive studies support this belief (Martin, 2001).

One study reported by Provine (2000a) found that participants who watched a humorous video while having their hands in ice water could endure the pain. The funnier they perceived the video, the longer they could endure the pain. The control group in this study viewed a documentary. The control group experienced the same amount of pain relief. This finding led to the conclusion that distraction, or a related cognitive process, contributed to the pain relief.

In a field study involving 26 females diagnosed with rheumatoid arthritis, researchers found that there was a significant decrease in self-reported pain ratings after watching a 1-hour performance of rakugo, a form of Japanese humor. Another small study of elderly residents in a long-term care facility indicated that the amount of pain medication used to manage their chronic pain decreased after watching a comedy.

Leise (1993) conducted a study of 30 women between the ages of 33 and 66 who had a diagnosis of rheumatoid arthritis and no other chronic problems. The study examined the relationship between chronic pain and a healthy sense of humor. Individuals who reported a high level of pain also reported using humor frequently. Leise (1993) noted that individuals who experience a lot of pain may need a lot of humor in their lives to cope with the stress of their pain. This study did not indicate that humor helped control the pain, however.

A study conducted by RxLaughter in collaboration with The National Cancer Institute in Thailand and Yale University School of Epidemiology and Public Health, looked at the effects of integration of funny Thai films and television shows into a support group for cancer survivors (Bhosai, Miwa & Hilber, 2007). The aim of this study was to determine if humor affects self-reported levels of pain, comfort and quality of life. Prior to the beginning of the study, the intervention group reported higher levels of pain and anxiety, lower levels of comfort and satisfaction, and more difficulty sleeping than the control group. The group that viewed 2 hours of humorous videos twice a day had decreased pain and anxiety, less difficulty sleeping, and higher levels of comfort and satisfaction, whereas the control group had no change.

This was a pilot study and there are questions left to answer. There is a question as to whether the improved scores for the therapy group are based on the intervention, or are a factor of time. Does the ability to cope with the disease over time affect the results seen, or is it really the treatment? Does the intervention group really receive less pain medication at night? This aspect was not explored. Since the intervention group reported improved levels of satisfaction with the care, the question is whether the level of satisfaction is based on viewing the films, or is there an increase in interaction that could be affecting satisfaction levels? Whatever it is, one thing the pilot study demonstrated, viewing humorous films offered physical signs of improvement.

There are some studies that looked at the use of humor during painful or uncomfortable interventions. The summation of these studies is that having a sense of humor trait is more beneficial than an induced humor state, and it appears that laughter's benefit to pain management is its ability to cause relaxation or distraction (Mahony, Burroughs, & Hieatt, 2001).

Mahony and colleagues (2001) became interested in discovering if expectation of the benefit from laughter or from relaxation would have an effect on pain threshold. All the participants except the control group were told that the video they would be watching would either increase or decrease their sensitivity to the discomfort caused by an inflated blood pressure cuff. This small study indicated that an induced humor state is no more effective than induced relaxation when it comes to coping with discomfort. The researchers do say that "it is fairly safe to assume that most people in pain would prefer a laughter intervention, particularly one of their own choosing, over relaxation exercises, hypnotism, or reading a brochure arguing the benefits of a particular program" (p. 17). More studies are needed.

Another small study revealed that patients who viewed comedy took lower doses of minor pain medication than those who watched action/adventure videos. Those given a choice of comedy videos needed lower doses of medication than those who did not have a choice. Those given a choice of action videos showed no effect of choice. This study indicates that humor preference is individual and that few things are as irritating as exposure to material that does not appear to be funny to that individual (Mahoney et. al, 2001).

The UCLA Children's Hospital has started a program in conjunction with Rx Laughter to try and ease sick children through multiple medical procedures and minimize the traumatic effects the children experience (Rx Laughter, 2002). The mission statement for Rx Laughter notes that it is a therapeutic nonprofit corporation involved in entertainment research, and education: "that continually strives to help children and adults who are suffering from the effects of physical and mental illness, by prescribing funny films and television shows as an important part of treatment care." The UCLA program is a collaboration between pediatrics, psychiatry, and the entertainment industry. As well as offering a diversion for children, this program looks at the behaviors and thoughts generated by the laughter. One area of interest is the relationship between humor, laughter, pain perception, and pain tolerance.

A study published in 2007 shares the effects of the study (Stuber, Hilber, Mintzer, Castaneda, Glover, & Zeltzer, 2009). This study looked at pain tolerance after immersing a child's hand in cold water. What they found was the intensity of the pain was rated the same each time, but the children were able to leave their hands in the cold water longer while watching the clips than either of the previous trials. The researchers concluded that watching funny videos increased the tolerance to moderately painful stimulus, but that the tolerance was not associated with a decrease in pain severity. Also, the number of times the child laughed was not associated with either pain severity or pain tolerance. This was a pilot study with a number of limitations. Further studies are needed to determine if watching funny videos is a viable option for increasing pain tolerance in children.

This next story by Dr. Hunter "Patch" Adams describes an experience he had that demonstrates how laughter and humor can affect pain reaction. Dr. Adams has been taking a group of therapeutic clowns to other countries as a way of trying to improve relations between those countries and the United States, to spread cheer and to offer a seminar in clowning for beginners and professional clowns (Adams, 1993). For 7 years he had taken a group to Moscow and St. Petersburg. One year he decided to add Estonia to the itinerary. They walked into a burn hospital and he noticed a woman standing outside a closed door crying. His knowledge and instinct told him this mother was agonizing over a very ill child. He knew clowning would not be appropriate with the mother but felt that clowning with the child might be helpful for both of them. He walked into the room dressed in full clown clothes to find a female doctor and her two female assistants starting a dressing change on a 5-year-old boy with third-degree burns over 60% of his body. He was "struck" by the lack of supplies, including strong pain medication, gloves, gowns, and masks.

The young boy, Radio, screamed with each tug of the dressing. Radio could not see Adams because of the position of the boy's neck, but when the team took a break, Adams walked over to the head of the bed and bent down. Radio looked at him and said, "You look beautiful." Adams stayed at the head of the bed smiling and laughing and talking with Radio during the rest of the dressing change. Radio did not scream again as the dressing change continued.

Adams mentions that he does not know what the catalyst was that resulted in the rest of the dressing change to appear to be pain free. He says, "Was it the sparkle in my eye, the duck hat on my head, the soothing stroking of his head, the words of love and encouragement – or was it simply skilled diversion?" We will never know the exact mechanism, but whatever it was, the rest of the dressing change appeared to be pain free.

SUMMARY

Although many studies are controversial because of limited sample sizes and research methodologies, there is evidence that humor positively affects the immune response. Studies also show that humor affects the cardiac and respiratory systems. Some positive correlations between pain management and the use of humor therapy also exist. Many studies have measured the physiological effects of humor and laughter, but more research is needed.

Lessons from this chapter:

- Physiological changes definitely occur.
- Humor triggers increases in immunoglobulins and killer T cells.
- Humor decreases cortisol levels.
- How effective these immunological changes are is not known.
- Endorphin release with humor is still not proven.
- Humor shows ability to help the cardiovascular and respiratory systems.
- Laughter during a painful procedure might increase tolerance for pain.
- There is some mechanism activated by humor that assists with pain control. What that mechanism is, is still not known.

EXAM QUESTIONS

CHAPTER 7
Questions 52-58

Note: Choose the one option that BEST answers each question.

52. The body's physiological response during acute stress is

    a. reduced secretion of cortisol.

    b. reduced heart rate and blood pressure.

    c. suppression of epinephrine.

    d. increased secretion of cortisol.

53. Humor increases the level of

    a. adrenocorticotropic hormone.

    b. dehydroepiandrosterone.

    c. immunoglobulin A.

    d. norepinephrine.

54. The immunoglobulin that increases with humor and is responsible for producing long-term immunity is

    a. IgA.

    b. IgG.

    c. IgM.

    d. IgB.

55. Laughter may be one way to improve respiratory function after surgery because it

    a. decreases pulmonary ventilation.

    b. relaxes chest and abdominal muscles.

    c. triggers a bellows action on the thoracic cavity.

    d. decreases oxygen saturation.

56. The results of Lebowitz studies (2002) indicate that when caring for patients with chronic obstructive pulmonary disease, nurses should use humor that leads to laughter

    a. as often as possible.

    b. cautiously.

    c. never.

    d. periodically.

57. The physiological process by which pain is reduced with humor is

    a. increased endorphins in the blood.

    b. improved levels of immunoglobulins.

    c. still unkown.

    d. strictly distraction.

58. According to one study cited by Mahony (2001), when patients were given a choice of the comedy videos they wanted to watch, their need for pain medication

    a. increased.

    b. decreased.

    c. stayed the same.

    d. varied.

CHAPTER 8

HUMOR AS A MODERATOR IN CANCER AND OTHER LIFE-THREATENING ILLNESSES

CHAPTER OBJECTIVES

After completing this chapter the reader will be able to discuss how humor can be helpful to individuals with cancer and other life-threatening illnesses.

LEARNING OBJECTIVES

After studying this chapter, the reader will be able to

1. explain how humor can assist in coping with breast cancer.

2. discern when, in the process of adjusting to a life-threatening disease, humor might be accepted.

3. discuss the efficacy of humor in end-of-life care.

4. design humor interventions to help patients with life-threatening diseases.

INTRODUCTION

"Laughter gives us distance. It allows us to step back from an event, deal with it and then move on."
— *Bob Newhart*

The diagnosis of cancer and other life-threatening illnesses causes feelings of fear and anxiety. Finding ways to decrease the emotional distress accompanying diagnosis is important. Humor is one method implicated as effective in assisting individuals to cope with the experience of cancer and other disease processes. This chapter will discuss how individuals with life-threatening diseases view humor as a coping mechanism. Much of the research that has been done involves patients with cancer. In addition, the author of the text conducted extensive interviews with 11 breast cancer patients and some of their stories will be shared.

The reason for the importance of understanding the impact of humor for people diagnosed with life-threatening illness is illustrated by a small study reported by Joshua, Cotroneo, and Clarke (2005) with terminally ill individuals. They all had a prognosis of about 6 months to live at the time of the interviews. Eighty-five percent responded that humor would be useful during their present situation; however, only 14% described any type of humor in their lives. Every individual indicated that humor was an important mechanism for social bonding. About 64% felt that humor helped them alter their perceptions of the situation that would otherwise be overwhelming. One aspect that enabled them to face the realities of everyday life was that of hope, as evidenced by 85% of the participants saying that humor gave them a sense of hope. The sad part is that many people, professional and nonprofessional alike, are hesitant to use humor with people deemed "terminally ill." If those of us in health care were to add humor to our plan of care maybe we could help the patient find that little ray of hope.

The learner must keep in mind that stories cannot be generalized to the whole population of people with cancer or other life-threatening diseases. However, a review of different stories told by individuals dealing with cancer and other life-threatening diseases indicates that humor is a mechanism that is employed to try to cope with the feelings, thoughts, and issues presented with a life-threatening illness.

CANCER, HUMOR, AND COPING

Once the diagnosis of cancer has been made, dealing with the treatment, potential disfigurement, pain, and everyday tension of knowing that one has a potentially fatal disease leads to stress and the need to develop mechanisms to deal with the feelings and thoughts that result. This process can be arduous because the fear of the unknown invades what the person perceived as his or her normal world before the diagnosis. The human mind can only handle so much fear and uncertainty, which is probably why the first process in dealing with such a diagnosis is denial. Eventually, the person begins to develop or tap into their usual coping strategies. One of the strategies that appear to be effective is the use of humor (Wikliniski, 1994; Johnson, 2002; Schwartz, 2006). Cancer patients reported that humor was an important element in helping them deal with their illness. Laughter helps cancer patients escape from the fears of pain, disfigurement, and potential death. Humor helps patients connect with others who are important in their lives.

An example is Sally who was diagnosed with breast cancer and was receiving chemotherapy. When she knew she was going to lose her hair, she went to her hairdresser. She said she wanted to have her head shaved. The first thing the hairdresser did was give her a Mohawk and they took pictures. This lightened the mood. The appointment had started out seriously, but when they took out the camera, they started to have fun. Soon after that day, when the stubble began to fall out, she thought it would be difficult for her and her daughters to deal with. Once again, she decided to have some fun. She took out two of her leg shavers, got her two daughters, sat on a towel on the floor of the bathroom, and her daughters shaved her head. They all had a great time laughing and joking, and her daughters felt they were helping their mom with her cancer (Schwartz, 2006).

As noted in the story above, not only does the individual diagnosed with cancer deal with issues of life and death, so does his or her family. Incorporation of humor is helpful for family members also. Interestingly, Sally, found that she and her daughters could use humor easily, but her husband had a very difficult time dealing with Sally's humor until he knew that she was going to survive (Schwartz, 2006).

Dr. Susan Love (1991), author of a well-known book on breast cancer, stated, "Some of my patients found that laughter is an important part of their healing process" (p. 335). A study by Carver et al. (1993) followed women with stage 1 and stage 2 breast cancer from pre-surgery to 1 year after surgery. The study found the use of humor was linked to lower levels of emotional distress. This was especially true at 3 months and 6 months, but did not seem to be true at 12 months. This trend might be because at 12 months the survivors had adapted to being a cancer survivor and the fear of dying was not as strong.

Wiklinski (1994) conducted a study using interviews and storytelling with five individuals diagnosed with cancer. Her desire was to discover if humor had meaning for persons adapting to a cancer experience. The participants had all completed a series of radiation and chemotherapy. One person was scheduled for a bone marrow transplant. All participants felt they had successfully adapted to the turmoil created by diagnosis and treatment. All the participants in this study indi-

"The doctor will be a little late...why don't you discuss each other's ailments until he gets here!"

Note. From DansCartoons.com. Used with permission.

cated that humor was one of the factors that helped them to adapt in a positive manner to their disease. However, they all shared that they needed to deal with the disease and accept "all the major things" before they were open to humor, joy, hope, peace, and feeling "up." The participants of this study indicated that humor helped them cope with fear, anger, frustration, and grief.

In 2006, a study by Schwartz looked at coping and humor usage in women with breast cancer. All the women were within 6 months of diagnosis. This is a critical time of adjustment for most cancer survivors. The following themes concerning humor usage emerged from her study: timing, physical transformation, emotional transformation, and connecting.

There were times when humor was not appreciated, especially when the person was feeling a high level of anxiety and fear. Physical transformation had to do with a sense of decreasing heaviness of the situation, or a sense of being physically lighter once the participant was able to use humor. All the participants also felt that humor was an important aspect for maintaining health. Humor also led to an affirmation that they were going to live, that physically they would survive this experience. Emotional transformation referred to concepts

such as changing perspective, relieving tension, and emotionally distancing themselves from the process. The last theme, that of connecting, has two components: the connection between people that humor facilitates, and the use of humor by the participants as a means of helping others decrease feelings of discomfort when interacting.

Reading some of the participant's stories might help the learner understand the significance of the four themes described above.

Timing

The level of fear that was experienced by the different women had a big effect on when they were able to start using humor as a coping mechanism. The higher the fear factor, the harder it was to appreciate others' use of humor and the more difficult it was to use humor themselves. Because all of the women claimed to use humor as a coping mechanism prior to diagnosis, the main issue with timing appeared to be associated with the level of fear experienced. It was not until their anxiety level decreased, usually because they saw things happening, such as surgery or the beginning of chemotherapy or radiation, that they were able to see humor in any of life's events.

As one person said:

"Even things you would (find funny) are not funny. They're almost offensive at times... especially in movies or on TV, they'll have humorous things about death and dying, and it was offensive then. It's not funny, it is just not funny. And I don't feel that way so much anymore. It's not meant to be offensive, but at the time it was."

Another shared that she made a deliberate decision to incorporate humor in her recovery almost right away. She shared:

"It isn't the very first day (laughter)...I went to the surgeon, he had the mammogram, he did the breast exam and he sent me from there to have a needle biopsy. I was pretty certain in that brief 45 minutes that I had breast cancer. I mean I was very convinced because of his urgency. Then they did it and the pathologist came right in and told me. Um, so the next day I went back to the surgeon because of him telling me these are the options and so forth, there is a little tiny bit of humor that day, although I was crying. I remember sitting on the table crying. Then he did say about losing my hair, that's when I started crying harder. Oh no, I forgot all about that. Then he did say something about the Sinead O'Connor look, I did chuckle about that, so he tried humor. But by the next day, or later that same day, I think that humor was already starting to come into it. I pretty much made up my mind, and I told another friend and he said he never saw anyone being so deliberate about this, but I did. I said to myself, you know what Kim, you've got to decide right now how you're going to be about this. It's a trick, you can be grumpy, and you can be out-of-sorts, and you can feel sorry for yourself. I can remember I was standing in my bedroom at the foot of my bed, and I said to myself I am going to have to decide what kind of person I'm going to be about this. You know, am I going to be grumpy, am I going to be feeling sorry for myself, am I going to make everyone miserable around me because I have had some misfortune or am I going to take it in stride and am I going to lead by example to be the same as I always am, only have breast cancer. There wasn't a choice when I put it to myself like that because who wants to be a grumpy old mess, you know. Pretty much at that point, I just shed all of my feeling sorry for myself and why me, and was it something I did to myself. Because, I mean, even my surgeon told me that cancer is the most nondiscriminatory disease there is, it hits everybody and/or anybody. So don't start sitting there thinking you are the lucky one that got picked. It doesn't have anything to do with you. Someone is going to get cancer and it happened to be you. I thought that was a really good way of putting it, too. Then I started thinking that what if I did this, I smoked for about twenty years, I thought oh, oh, that is my pun-

ishment. You know, all that kind of stuff. I just put all those thoughts aside and I said there's no reason to cry over spilled milk, I have breast cancer and now, what do I do about it, and off I went. I just think the humor started right in there."

There are a number of messages in the above comment. A person can make a choice, even when the situation can feel overwhelming. Here was an individual who deliberately chose to find a way to make the situation seem less overpowering by taking control and finding things to laugh about, or at least find humorous. And, she came to this decision almost right away. She was less incapacitated by the diagnosis than others who were interviewed. She also had a physician who was comfortable enough to try to use some subtle humor. With this patient, it worked. It might not have worked and then he could let it go. He also sized up the situation and realized that this patient might be ready to hear that cancer was indiscriminate and get the message that she was not to blame for having this disease. Being able to 'read' the patient is a skill that can help the patient put things in perspective.

Physical Transformation

The theme of physical transformation had to do with humor helping the person feel as if a large weight had been lifted. Although most of the time participants referred to the emotional burden of diagnosis and dealing with cancer, there were times when they had a sense of a physical heaviness. Sometimes the heaviness was tension within the person, and sometimes it was tension between people. Humor and laughter seemed to lift that heaviness or relieve the tension. As one person said, "A good hearty laugh just takes the burden off of you. You feel lighter afterwards. Physically, you just feel it."

One lady mentioned that when you feel good, when you're happy, "it's almost like you stand up straighter and you don't have that heaviness in your chest." Another lady referred to sadness as a heavy weight. She went on to say, "Humor lightens that heavy weight…That sad feeling makes me really sick."

The theme of life-affirmation is explained by one person this way, "Any time you can laugh about something funny, every time I can, it makes me feel more like I'm in the human race, more like I'm going to live; I can laugh, I can live." That aspect of being able to laugh, in finding humor in everyday aspects of life, confirming that the person is still alive has been shared by authors who have told their own stories about their cancer experience, as well as some of the literature on end-of-life issues reminding caregivers that being solemn about the dying person reminds them they are dying, whereas using humor tends to remind them they are still alive.

One woman who was dealing with a number of different disease processes shared that laughter reminded her that life could be enjoyable, even if she were in pain. "There are funny stories and I laugh because it brings such fulfillment to me. You know, that life can be so enjoyable in the midst of all this pain. I honestly never thought about laughter at all, and now, I honestly think it has helped save my life."

Emotional Transformation

The theme of emotional transformation included sub-themes of transcending, lightening, and distancing. Wiklinski (1994), in her study with cancer patients, referred to transcending as a way of opening new possibilities for envisioning one's life. Five of the participants in Schwartz's study mentioned that humor helped by changing or allowing them to put things in perspective. One person stated that humor helped her see that cancer was "not the end of the world." Another noted that humor "washes away the sadness." Another said that humor helped change focus and helped "a person realize that maybe it was not as grim as you thought it was." This person added that the change in focus might help the person think of another solution. One person mentioned that humor could

always change her perspective. This person wrote in her diary that participants were asked to keep.

There is more to laughter than laughing. Release, spontaneity, relaxation. A renewed mind. A lighter heart, a lighter mindset, a different perspective on the moment. A reminder of the fact that everything didn't used to be so overwhelming, serious, and that better days will come. Laughter refocuses my thought from me and from the heaviness of the situation.

The sub-theme of lightening referred to humor or laughter causing the sense of feeling emotionally lighter, less 'gloomy.' Some of the comments made regarding lightness related to humor follow:

- It lifts you up.

- It lightens the situation.

- With my funny humor it has lightened up the really devastating aspects of cancer.

- I don't feel as if I'm constrained or bound by things.

- It keeps you out of that dark place.

Distancing was chosen as a sub-theme because of comments by participants who mentioned that humor helped them cope by allowing them to distance themselves from the experience. One person shared that laughter allowed her to disassociate from the experience. She commented that laughter helped her cope by making it "like it is somebody else."

Distancing was also an issue when they felt that fear, anxiety, sadness, and depression distanced them from their ability to use and appreciate humor. One of the participants started to cry when she shared with the researcher how much she appreciated being able to laugh again. She claimed the tears were from relief and happiness.

Connecting

The last theme, that of connecting, had to deal with how humor helped the study participants connect with others. When a person is diagnosed with cancer, or any life-threatening disease, everyone in their family or social circle is also affected. Participants in the study found that humor helped form a connection and decrease tension between them and others. Humor initiated by the participants allowed others to relax and start laughing and telling jokes. Some of the study participants shared that it was hard to find humor or something to laugh at when they were alone. Humor was seen as needing to be shared.

An aspect of connecting was that of helping others. Many participants found that humor helped others cope or feel more relaxed. People tended to become tense when they found out the other person had cancer. The participants realized that people did not know what to say. Saying or doing something humorous seemed to decrease the other person's discomfort and gave that person permission to joke also. The following is just one story of how a cancer survivor used humor to help others. This situation occurred at work:

It was a big joke, but when I first lost my hair, the big thing was, you know the bald head, so we were playing around and having a good time, so she took a permanent marker and drew a face on the back of my head. Well, I went to my DARE officer in school and I said, 'J, look what she did. You know, you need to arrest her because she defaced public property, or private property rather.' So she went in and arrested her for defacing private property. And from there it went to a reprimand, a fake reprimand from our supervisor, ah, our superintendent for this whole thing. I gave S. (her boss) a Mr. Potato Head for the times when she needed to play with a bald head. And I gave her a coloring book, for when she wanted to be creative, she could color. And I gave her a sketch pad so that when she wanted to be creative but didn't want to stay inside those lines, she could draw all

those faces she wanted to draw on the sketch pad. And I gave her some washable ink so if she just couldn't help herself, she could draw on my head if she really wanted to. (laughter)

Another aspect of helping others was the concern participants had for their family members. One person said she did not want to be the reason others felt sad, so she tried to be happy when she was around her family. If she could not "put on a happy face" she would isolate herself. One of the women with children said she did not want her children to remember her sickly and sad. She stated:

There is a time and place for seriousness, especially with cancer, because it is serious. But to stay within the realm of seriousness for great lengths of time just adds cancer to cancer. I encourage myself and uplift my family when I can laugh.

This cartoon is a reminder that cancer, with all of its negatives, can have a humorous side.

Note. From BuckCash.com. Used with permission.

Most of the studies concerning coping, humor and cancer have been conducted using an adult population. There are two dissertations that have been done on children with cancer and the use of humor coping (Dowling, 2000; Le Vieux, 2002).

Dowling looked at sense of humor and its moderating effects on cancer stressors and psychosocial adjustment to cancer, immune function, and infection in school-age children. The results of this study indicated that children with a high sense of humor demonstrate a greater psychological adjustment despite the amount of cancer stressors. Also, the study revealed that coping humor had a positive effect on psychosocial adjustment to the daily hassles of living with cancer. There was also a strong correlation between high coping humor and decreased infections.

In the study by Le Vieux, the children stated that they needed time to adjust to the cancer diagnosis and that nothing seemed funny. What they wanted most was to be with their family, and to have time alone to adjust to the diagnosis. They all wanted, and sought, information about their disease process. The more they learned, the better or more in control they felt. When it came to hearing difficult or distressing information, they did want others to use humor with them.

The children in the Le Vieux study did use humor to cope with the body changes that occurred. Acceptance from peers is very important, and many of the participants shared that they joked with their friends about the hair loss. Some of their friends shaved their heads as a way of supporting the child with cancer. The participants of this study also joked and teased with their doctors, nurses, and other staff members when they had treatment. However, there had to have been a good relationship developed before they were comfortable being playful or using humor with their healthcare providers.

Le Vieux looked at the difference between the children's relationships and humor usage with family and friends versus their use of humor with other children with cancer and with healthcare and camp staff. Most of the children attended a camp for children with cancer. When the study participants were with other children who had cancer, whether it be in the hospital or at camp, they tended to use humor and playfulness as a way of connecting with one another. They also used humor and teasing with the staff caring for them. They tended to use playful pranks with the medical staff. The children in this study indicated that humor may alleviate symptoms, promote positive feelings, build rapport, and facilitate learning, but it was most important that they get straight, honest, and clear answers to their concerns. Important information from this study is that a trusting relationship must be developed with healthcare personnel, parents, and teachers before humor can be accepted by the child.

HUMOR AND OTHER LIFE-THREATENING DISEASES

There is little research in the use of humor with other life-threatening diseases. However, it seems that people with other life-threatening diseases do use humor as part of their attempts to moderate the devastating emotional effects of disease. It makes sense that anyone under a lot of stress would find humor a means of changing perspective, taking a break from the anxiety and fears of dealing with severe disease processes.

Eddy Sakowicz (2007), a young man in Kentucky who is dealing with kidney failure, shares his story of devastation from the disease and rebuilding with humor on the Renal Support Network (RSN) Web site. He was diagnosed with kidney failure in his late 20s while working on a master's degree. He found that his friends stopped laughing and seemed to turn away. He states,

> *They thought this was no time for me to joke, but a time to grow up and be responsible. Months went by, and no laughter, only pills, doctors, and the harmonious beep-beep of the machines. I felt fragile, and worst of all, sick.*

He continued to share how he got tired of the silence and decided to go to a party where some of his friends were. His friends were outside and some of them were smoking. Eddy turned to one of his friends and sarcastically stated, "You know smoking rots your lungs!" Whereby his friend turned to him and said, "You know nagging rots your kidneys!" After a stunned silence, Eddy began to laugh. He states, "Suddenly, from the center of my deepest sorrows came out the loudest belly laugh." That laugh gave his friends permission to laugh and suddenly the world did not seem so gloomy. Eddy explains how that laughter caused him to feel. "I realized what it felt like to be alive, to once again laugh and release all that was hurting."

Once again we see how important humor may be to someone facing serious illness. The aspect of feeling as if his world had come to an end is apparent in the sharing of Eddy's experience. The ability to laugh again made a difference in how he perceived his illness and his life. He goes on to say, "Life began to regain its excitement, and I realized that at 'pity parties' you never get good presents. That one good belly laugh made me feel human again."

It doesn't seem to matter if the disease is cancer, kidney failure, multiple sclerosis, AIDS, or any other life-threatening disease, humor is an important part of coping with the illness. As healthcare providers, it is our responsibility to recognize the need to laugh, and to help our patients/clients and their families find ways to enjoy life and decrease the effects of living with a life-threatening, debilitating disease.

HUMOR AND DYING

Some people think that humor has no place in the dying process. Alan Klein (1998) tried to dispel that myth in his book *Courage to Laugh*. He talked to people who were dying and people who were bereaved and compiled their stories about humor and coping. The result is a book that is filled with examples of how people can take charge of the dying process or the bereavement over loss of a

loved one and use humor to lighten the grief or the pain of loss.

Part of the problem with exploring the use of humor during the care of the terminally ill involves American culture's avoidance of and discomfort with death. Death is considered a solemn affair. However, if a person is dying, does he or she really want to be sad and solemn all the time? What about the belief that life is to be lived until death? Yes, pain and deterioration may occur during the dying process; however, humor can still be employed to try to offer a period of relief.

Hospice nurses Graham and Cates (cited in Herth, 1995) suggest that humor provides care for the whole person, something that is now known to be important in health care. Humor encourages expression of a range of emotions, helps facilitate coping with pain and loss, and helps provide a way of framing life even if life is limited (Herth, 1995). Branum (1990, cited in Herth, 1995) believes 'that humor provides a momentary escape into a place of freedom and power' (p. 219). This can be a wonderful gift to someone who has a sense of powerlessness.

Herth (1995) conducted a study that involved 14 terminally ill adults. Many of them expressed that sharing something positive made them feel like "a real person again" (Herth, 1995, p. 220). Most expressed a sentiment that has also been expressed by cancer patients: Humor allowed them to see things in a more positive manner and put a new light on their situations. Several of the patients felt that the constant seriousness of their present situation made them feel isolated "and as if they were already dead" (Herth, 1995, p. 220). The participants felt that humor enhanced and enriched their lives even though their time on earth was limited.

Because dying is serious business, it might be up to the nurse to send signals that tell the patient that it is okay to laugh. Once people sense that humor is okay, they are more likely to share and bring forth their own humor potential. When dealing with the dying, it is important to allow room for all ranges of emotion; too much humor, like too much crying, can wear on the patient.

IMPLICATIONS FOR CARE

What can healthcare providers do to assist individuals in their quest for coping with disease processes? How can healthcare providers effectively, and sensitively, add levity to the seriousness of dealing with life-threatening diseases? There are a few suggestions offered here that can be used to assist those dealing with life-threatening disease processes in finding humor as an alternative and moderator for the overwhelming feelings they may be experiencing.

First and most important, be sensitive. What is important to incorporate is therapeutic humor, humor that works as complimentary "medicine" to assist the patient or client to find a way to deal with his or her disease process. This is not a case of being funny, or telling jokes, or even being playful just for the sake of making the other person laugh. It is a case of sensitively adding a little levity into a difficult situation so that the other person will feel less tense, less overwhelmed, and more able to deal with the present situation.

To be sensitive you need to understand what phase of adjustment the person is experiencing. If they are very tense, angry, or scared, humor might not be appropriate. This would be the time to listen and encourage them to express those negative feelings. Then, saying something with a hint of humor that is not meant to be offensive, might be just the thing that they need to 'lighten-up." In order to add humor, rapport must be established. Listen carefully to what the patient has to say. By listening carefully the healthcare provider might pick up on a statement and make a comment that would be enough to cause a smile.

The healthcare provider should approach everyone with a smile. Not a silly grin, but a genuine, kind smile. When someone smiles they do not seem as formidable. Do not be afraid to smile at the patient, even one who seems depressed. A kind smile goes a long way, and says I am glad to see you.

A patient was lying in bed after having a mastectomy with TRAM flap reconstruction surgery. Because the fat from her abdomen had been used, she had an abdominal wound as well as the breast wound. Her plastic surgeon visited her the day after surgery. She was in pain, depressed over losing her breast, worried about her future and, overall, not feeling well. He checked her breast and said everything looked good. Then, as he was getting ready to leave, he looked at the patient and said, 'You have to remember, I took the fat from your abdomen and moved it to your breast area. That fat is abdominal fat so if you tend to gain weight in your abdomen and are not careful, you will start walking like this," and he proceeded to walk lopsided. The patient couldn't help but laugh, even though her abdomen was sore when she did. The laughter lightened her mood, and 16 years later she still vividly remembers that experience, and it still brings a smile to her face (personal experience, Schwartz).

Being sensitive also means being careful with comments, jokes or puns. Humor can be hurtful as well as helpful. Sarcastic comments, sexual or sexist jokes, religious jokes, humor that puts others down, or gallows humor are inappropriate. Gallows humor is the type of humor that is used by some professions that deals with the pain, suffering, and death they may deal with frequently, but it is seen as cruel and hurtful to others.

Helping people who are ill and/or dying find a way to be playful helps add humor to their lives.

An elderly woman in a nursing home knew she was near death. After all, she was an ill 82-year-old. She was depressed and had not eaten much in the past 48 hours. The nurse walked into her room and sat down to talk with her.

The lady looked up and said, "You know, I've done a lot of things in my life, but I have had one dream I never got to fulfill, and now I'm dying."

The nurse took her hand and asked, "What is that dream?"

"I've always wanted to go to Hawaii."

At this point in the woman's life, going to Hawaii was not possible. However, the nurse encouraged her to share what she thought going to Hawaii would be like. When she finished sharing, her mood was lighter. The nurse smiled at her and said, "We can't take you to Hawaii, but we will bring Hawaii to you." With suggestions from the resident, the nursing home staff planned a luau. Everyone was invited, the dining hall was decorated with Hawaiian décor, the local florist donated flowers, a pig was roasted, the local dance studio had young girls come and dance Hawaiian dances, and everyone had a great time. There were many laughs shared and for the next 2 weeks of the woman's life, she would smile and talk about her "trip" to Hawaii.

A few of the women interviewed by Schwartz mentioned that sharing about humor caused them to be more aware of humor in their lives. It is possible that, just asking about coping mechanisms they are presently using to deal with their illness, and specifically if humor is a part of their coping, is a way of making people more aware of humor's potential.

Take a humor inventory. Ask the person if they use humor, or have used it in the past. Ask them to share what things they find funny. What makes them laugh? Favorite comedian? Favorite sitcom? Pets? Children? Asking may be the key to reminding the person that there was a time life did not seem so overwhelming and it may be possible for that to happen again.

It is often easier to accept humor about a certain disease process when it comes from someone going through, or has gone through, the experience.

People who have had or presently have cancer can say or do things that are more accepted by others experiencing cancer. As an example: a newly diagnosed breast cancer patient attended a cancer support group for women. When her time came to share, she told her story and mentioned that she was trying to decide if she should have a lumpectomy or a mastectomy and, if she has the mastectomy, should she have reconstruction or not. Everyone in the room was seriously supportive and encouraging her to share and ask questions. She asked what the prosthesis was like. At that point, one of the older members of the group said 'Here, check this out," as she reached into the top of her shirt and pulled out her prosthesis, which she threw across the room to her. At that point, someone said, 'Oh, my, flying boobs," and everyone started to laugh (personal experience).

Engaging in humor and playfulness (which leads to smiles) can cause the healthcare provider to be vulnerable. If the healthcare provider is comfortable being a little vulnerable, it gives the patient or client the license to also be vulnerable. Find ways to put a little playfulness into the situation. This can be difficult since we have been programmed from childhood that we should be serious about problems. Many of us have heard our parents say things like, "wipe that smile off your face," or, "this is not a laughing matter, so stop laughing." As children, play comes easily, but as we get older we are told to act more mature, take responsibility, and be serious.

Clifford Kuhn, a psychiatry professor at the University of Louisville School of Medicine in Kentucky talks about the HaHaHa prescription (Kuhn, 2006). Before we can help our patients tap into their humor potential, it is important for the healthcare provider to be able to tap into their own humor potential.

Kuhn's first Ha is one of the most important ones: *humor attitude*. Kuhn states, "We have been taught that humor is for recreational purposes only.

Nobody has ever taught us that the way to become more effective and efficient when we are in the midst of a terrible problem is to lighten up" (Kuhn, 2006). Kuhn says the best way to reverse our thinking, and to help us recognize that humor does not mean we do not take our situation seriously, is to recognize there is a big difference between being funny and having fun. He advocates not worrying about being funny, but thinking of ways to have fun. He says having fun is "an attitude of willingness to look for the positive element in any situation, no matter how dire it is." He goes on to say that, if a person can get hold of that attitude, they can "discover that it's possible to have more fun anytime, anywhere."

The second Ha, according to Kuhn, is *humor aptitude.* That doesn't mean the ability to tell jokes or to be a funny person. It really means something very simple. Smile more and take yourself less seriously. Learn how to see the humor, and learn how to share it with sensitivity. When you work at taking yourself less seriously, humor tends to follow.

Here is an example of how humor just happens in the midst of a very frightening time.

Cliff Khun's daughter lost her first pregnancy. Six months later his daughter-in-law went into labor prematurely, delivering a baby who was underdeveloped and not breathing. The baby was in the intensive care unit "fighting for his life." Kuhn and his wife were "struggling with the fear, rage, and pain of a possible second heartbreak in less than a year" (Kuhn, 2003). The first time Kuhn and his wife were allowed to visit the baby in the intensive care unit they felt a lot of tension and fear. "The tension was made only worse by the presence of all the technology – the blinking lights, the electronic alarms, those huge machines supporting such tiny, frail bodies. It was a daunting moment" (p. 16).

As they walked to their grandson's bassinet, Kuhn's wife saw another baby under an ultraviolet light to control jaundice.

She grabbed Kuhn's arm and whispered, "What is that blue light?"

He recounts, "Without thinking, I just blurted out the first thing that came to mind. 'Sweetheart, that baby's on sale for the next ten minutes'" (p. 17).

Although, as Kuhn says, it was not very funny, it did help break the tension and helped to make the experience a little easier.

The third Ha is *humor action.* Kuhn says this is the last, and least important of the Has because, if you take care of the first two Has, this one will just happen. Some people think that this Ha means telling jokes or being funny, but what it really means is to be aware. Humor action means listening, saying thank you, being playful, and admitting your mistakes in a humorous manner.

Designing humor interventions can be as simple as having a humor basket or a shelf in the hallway with humorous books, comics, and a few humorous toys, to having a humor cart that volunteers can take around to share. Healthcare providers can wear silly buttons or neckties. One older woman had a pin that said, "The older I get, the better I was." When people read it the response was usually a comment and always a smile. When there is a sense that it would be OK to ask, find out what the person finds funny. If they say nothing is funny right now, ask if they used to laugh. If they say yes, find out what it was that they used to find funny. Most of all, remember that humor is not always welcome. Pay attention to the comments and behaviors of the patient, and go cautiously.

CASE STUDY

Marge, a 46-year-old college professor, was diagnosed with breast cancer. She was recently married to a coworker and had just moved into her new home. Life had been going well as she adjusted to her new life and the joys of a new marriage. The news of her breast cancer left her devas-

tated. How could this happen to her at a time like this? What would happen with this new marriage? Will he stick by her, or leave like her first husband, as soon as things got tough? Prior to her diagnosis she could be seen on campus smiling and joking with staff and students. After the diagnosis, nothing seemed funny. She became annoyed at others who tried to cheer her up, except when that person was her husband. She had her surgery and started chemotherapy. One day a coworker and she were talking about their reactions when they don't feel well. Her coworker vehemently said, 'When I'm sick with a cold or something, I get so impatient. It really pisses me off to have to deal with stuff like that." At that point, Marge started to laugh, a good strong belly laugh. She realized how much she missed having a good belly laugh, and how much better it made her feel. Marge shared, 'That was a turning point for me as I realized how much better it felt to smile and laugh. Although I have times when I'm scared or feel sorry for myself, my pity-parties have decreased in length. Humor helps me put my fears on a shelf for awhile."

Questions

1. What are the factors that might have prevented Marge from appreciating humor soon after diagnosis?

2. What might have been Marge's reaction if a healthcare provider had attempted to use humor with her in the early stage of adjustment to her diagnosis?

3. How could a healthcare provider determine if Marge was ready to accept humor as a means of coping with her illness?

4. What might have caused Marge's laughter when her coworker shared how she felt when a disease process slows her down?

Discussion

The level of fear experienced by Marge appears to be the factor most affecting her ability to utilize humor. Interestingly, her husband's attempt at humor is accepted, but no one else's attempt is appreciated. This might be based on the relationship between them, and/or the recognition that he is also dealing with fears and concerns and humor is one way he can cope.

Until her fear level decreases, humor attempted by the healthcare provider might be viewed as insensitive and uncaring. This, in turn, could lead to anger, increased anxiety, and frustration at the individual or even the entire healthcare system. When Marge is seen to smile or even share events in a humorous manner, the healthcare provider would have a clue that it might be OK to start introducing humor into their relationship. This can be done by saying something in a light-hearted manner or by talking to her about the use of humor as a coping mechanism.

One might never know what the actual trigger is that allows laughter to occur. In Marge's case with her coworker, it might have been the fact that Marge was dealing with a life-threatening disease, yet her coworker talked about her reaction to something as mundane as a cold. There is an element of incongruity to the situation. Incongruity is one of the main elements that is believed to cause a humorous reaction. It might also have been the realization of how upset and "pissed-off" Marge felt at having to deal with cancer when there was so much else she would rather be dealing with. Whatever it was, it was obviously time for Marge to start finding more effective ways to deal with her present situation. It has been said that the human brain can only handle so much stress before it will start trying to find a way to decrease the stress. Humor is often an effective way to do that.

SUMMARY

The main emphasis of this chapter is the use of humor in coping with life-threatening diseases, predominantly cancer. Cancer is the main emphasis because most of the research in this area has been done with cancer survivors, plus the research conducted by this author was on using humor to cope with breast cancer, making examples available to the learner. Dealing with life-threatening diseases causes high levels of anxiety and fear. Individuals' views of themselves, their life, and how they fit within society is challenged. Humor is one way to decrease the level of stress experienced.

The lessons from this chapter are:

- Humor is a useful tool in decreasing stress through
  - changing perspective,
  - allowing the person to dissociate from the problem for a brief period,
  - sharing with others,
  - offering some relief from intense emotions,
  - a sense of emotional and physical 'lightening."

- During periods of high levels of stress or fear, humor may not be appropriate.

- It is important to have a level of rapport developed before attempting humor in life-threatening situations.

- Modeling behavior, such as wearing a silly button or being playful, gives the patient permission do the same.

- Ask about a patient's use of humor as a coping mechanism.

- Be sensitive.

- Smile; it might make everyone wonder what you are up to, and it causes others to smile also.

- Although there may be a time humor is not appropriate, there almost always is a time when it is. Be alert for that time. Therapeutic humor can make life seem a lot less overwhelming, and that can help give the person the emotional strength they need to continue living, no matter how many hours, days, or years they may have left.

EXAM QUESTIONS

CHAPTER 8
Questions 59-65

Note: Choose the one option that BEST answers each question.

59. Humor during a life-threatening illness is an important mechanism to help patients

    a. cover up real feelings.

    b. deal with their illnesses.

    c. avoid discussing the diagnosis.

    d. keep the family engaged.

60. Research has shown that the use of humor presurgery and postsurgery for breast cancer is associated with

    a. lower levels of emotional distress.

    b. the patient not taking the diagnosis seriously.

    c. improved compliance with treatment.

    d. faster wound healing.

61. Before patients with life-threatening diagnoses can be open to humor, they must

    a. deal with the disease and accept "all the major things."

    b. determine treatment modalities.

    c. become knowledgeable about the diagnosis.

    d. complete the grieving process.

62. Research has shown that the time patients with life-threatening diagnoses can most commonly begin to use humor themselves is

    a. anytime depending on their personality.

    b. after psychological intervention.

    c. after the anxiety and fear levels decrease.

    d. when they are declared "cured."

63. When using humor with children who have a life-threatening diagnosis, it is important for the healthcare provider to

    a. avoid discussing their illness.

    b. refrain from mentioning any disfigurement.

    c. develop a relationship first.

    d. begin using humor as soon as possible after the diagnosis.

64. Humor is important in the dying process is because it

    a. encourages the expression of a range of emotions.

    b. helps the patient accept powerlessness.

    c. keeps the family distracted from the reality of death.

    d. has no arbitrary limits.

65. A strategy that might be helpful in using humor with a particular patient is to first

    a. poke fun at other patients.

    b. take the patient's "humor inventory."

    c. share a book of cartoons with the patient.

    d. collect funny stories about the patient from family members.

CHAPTER 9

THE USE OF HUMOR IN CRISES AND DISASTER SITUATIONS

If you can find humor in it, you can survive it.
— Bill Cosby

CHAPTER OBJECTIVES

After completing this chapter, the reader will be able to discuss the role of humor in crises and disaster situations and discern when healthcare provider intervention is most appropriate.

LEARNING OBJECTIVES

After studying this chapter, the reader will be able to

1. identify the psychological factors that affect humor reactions during crises.

2. list ways individuals have found to incorporate humor into their lives following a crisis.

3. explain the healthcare provider's role in crisis humor.

4. describe how humor helped prisoners of war (POWs) and other victims of war survive imprisonment and torture.

INTRODUCTION

Some people feel that humor is inappropriate during a crisis; however, others find that humor helps them put perspective on the crisis (Buxman, 2001; Frankl, 1963; Henman, 2001; Ritz, 1995; Sultanoff, 1995; Wooten & Dunkelblau, 2001). Ritz (1995) notes that a disaster occurs in the world every 8½ days. Now with the ongoing crisis in the Middle East, disasters seem to occur on an almost daily basis. It can be difficult for people to see any humor in a crisis. One crisis that almost every person in the United States can identify with occurred September 11, 2001. This chapter looks at how individuals resolved their experiences of September 11, as well as other crises such as the Holocaust, natural disasters, and being Prisoners of War (POWs).

SEPTEMBER 11

The tragedy that occurred on September 11, 2001 was so horrendous that it took a while before humor returned, even for those people who use humor as a coping mechanism. Klein (2001) notes that one news reporter stated it took 5 days, 2 hours, 8 minutes, and 1 second from the time the first plane hit the World Trade Center for the first attempts at humor to appear on the Internet. Buxman (2001), a registered nurse who presents humor and stress management workshops, notes that people mentioned they wanted to laugh but could not or were afraid to because of what others would think. Wooten and Dunkelblau (2001) note, "On September 11, Americans lost their will to laugh."

Sultanoff (1995) states that "during a crisis humor is often experienced and perceived by individuals immersed in the crisis as insensitive and even hurtful." He theorizes that individuals closest to the crisis are "more likely to integrate the crisis into their internal emotional being" (p. 2). Wooten and Dunkelblau (2001) explain that there is an inability to separate the inner emotional self from the emotional pain of the event. As distance from the crisis occurs, individuals are less likely to experience the merging of self with the crisis and are more able to experience humor aimed at the crisis.

The following story exemplifies how those involved in a crisis might be able to use humor.

A group of office workers at the World Trade Center were running down flight after flight of stairs, not knowing if they had the strength to continue. They reached the 11th floor feeling exhausted and as if they could not go on. Then one woman suggested they pretend it was New Year's Eve and start the countdown. En masse, they began a countdown with each flight of stairs and shouted out "10, 9, 8, 7, 6, 5, 4, 3, 2, 1." Encouraged by the levity, they all made it to the street and safety.

It was so difficult to find things to laugh at during the first few days following the attack on the World Trade Center that even Jay Leno had difficulty finding material to use. Comics were careful and cautious about what they said. News items that had appeared before September 11 became material for gags. Comics used opening lines such as, "Remember the good ole days of the West Nile virus?" Jay Leno got laughs with "America must now protect itself from angry religious extremists. But enough about Jerry Falwell."

DISASTER SITUATIONS

Sandra Ritz (1995) is a nurse who has studied survivor humor following disasters. Disasters include hurricanes, earthquakes, tornadoes, volcanic eruptions, floods, war, terrorist attacks, riots, radiation accidents, airplane crashes, multivehicle accidents, epidemics, or any number of unexpected natural or man-made catastrophes. When a healthcare provider deals with a disaster, flexibility and creativity are essential skills. The healthcare provider has little time to worry about what might be happening outside the immediate situation. What must have occurred for the healthcare providers involved in September 11, especially those who lived or worked near the World Trade Center?

Humor After a Disaster

As Ritz (1995) notes, the use of humor in a disaster situation can work as a coping strategy by relieving tension, managing stress, and reframing perspective. Sultanoff (1995) notes that humor provides a perspective and helps us deal with emotional turmoil.

As Jay Leno said following a California earthquake:

It's not all tragedy. You have to like the way the earthquake has brought this city together. I was driving down Sunset Boulevard and I noticed a white man, a black man, and a Hispanic man all looting together (Ritz, 1995, p. 198).

Gallows humor is the most common form of humor used in disaster situations. Ritz (1995) refers to gallows humor as "survivor humor." She states that "survivor humor is an active defense mechanism that helps to cope with threats and fears instead of surrendering to them" (p. 200). It may be difficult for those not directly affected by the disaster to understand the humor, but for the person affected, humor can be used to shock oneself out of horror and anxiety.

One example of survivor humor occurred during major widespread fires in California. In the neighborhoods where all of the homes were burned except for the fireplaces, people wore t-shirts that read: "My chimney is bigger than your chimney!" (Ritz, 1995, p. 200).

The Disaster Relief Act of 1974 recognized the mental health needs of those involved in disasters. "This act mandates that the National Institute of Mental Health provide mental health crisis counseling services and training as part of the disaster relief effort" (Ritz, 1995, p. 204). The biggest problems following a disaster are problems of living and readjustment. However, people are relatively resilient, and most people recover from the temporary emotional stress of a crisis. Grief reactions are also a common and normal part of a crisis or disaster. After all, a person experiences loss when his or her home is damaged or destroyed by fire, earthquake, or another natural disaster.

Three factors are essential in survivors' emotional recovery:

1. relief from stress;

2. talking about the experience;

3. passage of time

(Ritz , 1995).

We know humor is effective for stress relief; yet, until Ritz's (1995) study, there was very little research on the use of humor in disaster situations. The emphasis in the literature has been placed on the human service workers supporting usual coping mechanisms rather than looking at how humor might be utilized (Farberow & Fredrick, 1978, cited in Ritz, 1995). Humor assists in adaptation to change following a crisis and is an important element in long-term recovery for disaster survivors.

There are four emotional phases survivors experience after a disaster: heroic, honeymoon, disillusionment, and reconstruction. During the heroic phase, survival is the basic concern. The honeymoon phase occurs 1 week to 3 to 6 months after the disaster and involves recovery of optimism. The disillusionment phase occurs 2 months to 2 years after the disaster. During this phase, anger, resentment, and disappointment are common. The person

may feel oppressed by the agencies and organizations that have invaded the community. The reconstruction phase is a period of recovery, rebuilding, and acceptance (Ritz,1995).

As mentioned previously, passage of time helps heal those affected by a disaster. Leigh (2001) notes that humor tends to return as time passes and the distance from the crisis grows longer.

Different types of humor are prevalent during each of the emotional phases experienced after a disaster. Table 9-1 shows the types of humor that are commonly used during those phases.

TABLE 9-1: DISASTER PHASES AND HUMOR USAGE	
Phase	**Type of Humor used**
Heroic	Spontaneous
Honeymoon	Hopeful, reflects a sense of optimism
Disillusionment	Negative or sarcastic humor aimed at outside assistance
Reconstruction	Reflects a sense of community
(Ritz, 1995)	

During the heroic phase, humor is spontaneously produced by the survivor to relieve tension and overcome fear (Ritz, 1995). It might not be viewed as humorous to an outsider. The person or persons not directly affected by the crises might view humor used by the victims of the crisis as crude or strange or just not funny.

One example of humor during the heroic phase was shared by Ritz (cited in Klein, 1998): "Two hikers, caught on the coast trail of Kauai when Hurricane Iniki struck, sang the theme song from 'Gilligan's Island.' They kept up their spirits and dispelled their anxiety by reframing the situation in a comical format" (p. 161).

After Hurricane Katrina, the following sign was seen in one Mississippi yard where the house was completely blown away, "Looters will be shot on sight. At least we have some bullets left."

Most of the disaster-type humor occurs during the honeymoon phase. The humor during this phase is typically positive and hopeful. It reflects a sense of optimism. It usually lacks anger and assists in denial of negative emotions or difficulty. An example of this type of humor from the first example was a t-shirt that read, "Landscaped by Iniki" (Klein, 1998).

During the disillusionment phase, the type of humor that might be appropriate in earlier phases might now be misinterpreted because the survivors are feeling bitter. During the reconstruction phase, humor returns slowly. The humor might portray the disillusionment felt with the disaster assistance provided. During this phase, survivors commonly feel isolated, angry, and pessimistic. Survivor humor reflects these feelings. For example, after Hurricane Andrew hit the Florida coast, some people wore t-shirts that read, "I survived Hurricane Andrew, but FEMA [the Federal Emergency Management Agency] is killing me" (Klein, 1998, p. 161).

Six months following hurricane Katrina in 2005, t-shirts with the following sayings appeared in t-shirt shops that were still open: "I Stayed in New Orleans for Katrina and All I Got Was This Lousy T-Shirt, a New Cadillac and a Plasma TV," which reflected on the problems of looting. Another one that expressed the bitterness of the problems with the rescue effort read, "Where Is FEMA? Federal Employees Missing Again' (Weeks, 2006).

Another example of disillusionment humor occurred following Hurricane Iniki in 1992 in Kauai. This example demonstrates how language and cultural differences between survivors and relief workers can increase frustration and perhaps cause anger. A comedy skit on KONG radio went as follows:

Cheryl: Hi, I'm Cheryl from Cold-Hand Insurance Company. I'm here to look at your home. Are you Mrs. Kam-a-ka?"

Mrs. Ka maka: No, that's Mrs. Ka maka…Never mind girl, you call me Auntie…

Cheryl: Tell me, was there any damage done to your davenport, your living area, your veranda, your portecochére, or your daybed?

Mrs. Ka maka: No, but I had damage on top of my sofa, inside da parlor, da lanai, da garage, and on top of my pune'e (Pune'e is Hawaiian for couch or single bed.) (cited in Ritz, 1995, p. 201).

Reconstruction humor commonly reflects a sense of community as people begin to rebuild their lives. The humor seems to reflect collective goals, fears, problems, and a sense of acceptance plus adaptation to change. An example of this type of humor occurred after the multiple disasters that affected the southern California area. Residents were heard to remark, "Los Angeles has four distinct seasons: Earthquake, Flood, Firestorm, and Mud Slide" (Klein, 1998).

Karyn Buxman (2001) notes:

Nineteen ninety-three marked "the Flood of 500 Years" on the Mississippi River. Communities along the entire river experienced flooding, destruction of property, loss of homes and jobs, and sometimes death. Yet, humor marked the will of people to keep their spirits afloat, not to be oppressed and depressed by the Muddy Mississippi. In Iowa, the *Des Moines Register* held a contest, "I'm a Floody Mess," where contestants tried to one-up one another with descriptions of their misery. When the local water system failed as a result of the flood, and running water for drinking and bathing was no longer an option, one contestant wrote, "I smell so bad that my Sure deodorant is undecided." (p. 13)

After a major Midwest flood, the following billboards were spotted (cited in Klein, 1998):

Questions about the weather?
Call 1-800-NOAH

Welcome to Missouri,
The Row Me State
(Missouri is known as "The Show-Me State")

The weather lately gives a whole new meaning
to Roe vs. Wade

The above examples also point out the use of community resources (in this case, the media) in helping to support other members of the community. In a general disaster, having others in the situation who can understand the frustrations of the loss as well as the frustrations of dealing with disaster relief organizations helps survivors through the experience.

DISASTER WORKERS' RESPONSE

Research shows that many disaster and emergency workers have at least one symptom of post-traumatic stress disorder (PTSD). Training programs and simulation exercises aim at preventing disaster workers from experiencing stress in the first place (Ritz, 1995). Fortunately, organizations such as The Red Cross and The Pan American Health Organization now recognize humor as one of the important strategies for dealing with stress by those working at a disaster site (Stanhope & Lancaster, 2004).

Just as disaster survivors attempt to adapt and manage, so do disaster relief workers and other healthcare providers. Healthcare workers may be directly affected by being survivors or indirectly affected by needing to care for survivors. Disaster relief workers and healthcare workers giving care need effective methods of coping, just as those directly affected by the disaster do. Healthcare providers and disaster relief workers can use humor to decrease their own stress and connect with other members of the disaster relief team. Psychologist Paul McGhee (n.d.) has been told by people at FEMA conferences, state emergency response teams, and police, "If we didn't laugh at some of the things that happen, we'd never survive this job." Nurses, physicians, emergency medical technicians, and others who work in emergency departments, critical care units, and other units where life and death often hang in the balance have shared that they use black humor to survive.

Some of the jokes that people make after disasters may be interpreted as sick and inappropriate by others. For example, after an emergency response team spent the morning putting bodies from a plane crash in bags, someone said, "The bag lunches are here."

After the Delta crash in the 1980s, the following comments were heard for a number of years among relief workers:

At Delta, we now offer three classes of service: smoking, nonsmoking, and burned beyond recognition.

Delta now offers you free drinks if you present your dental records when purchasing your ticket.

Healthcare providers who work in disaster situations need to remember that humor can be helpful or hurtful. To use humor effectively, the provider must assess the survivor's current phase of recovery. The healthcare worker should also keep in mind that the humor appreciated by one person may be different from the humor appreciated by another, depending on what phase of adjustment the two individuals have reached. Inappropriate humor can be more hurtful than helpful. Assessing a patient's needs and survival phase is important in order to design or utilize appropriate humor. Being aware of which type of humor is appropriate for which phase of recovery is also important. Humor used therapeutically and judiciously can be helpful for the survivor. Learning to laugh again may be essential for emotional coping.

HUMOR WITH LOSS OF FREEDOM

Captain Gerald Coffee, a former Vietnam POW, shared in his book *Beyond Survival,* "Laughter sets the spirit free to move through even the most tragic circumstances. It helps us shake our heads clear, get our feet back under us and restore our sense of balance and purpose. Humor is integral to our peace of mind and ability to go beyond survival" (Coffee, 1990, p. 131).

In Coffee's place of captivity, an old cell had been converted into a shower. On the wall of the shower, the following message appeared: "Smile, you're on Candid Camera." Coffee (1990) states that when he saw this message, "I laughed out loud, enjoying not only the pure humor and incongruity of the situation, but also appreciating the beautiful guy who had mustered the moxie to rise above his own dejection and frustration and pain and guilt to inscribe a line of encouragement to those who would come after him…he deserved a medal for it." (pp. 131-132).

It is hard to imagine using humor to survive the Holocaust or to survive the tortures of being a POW during the Vietnam War. However, humor is one of the mechanisms people used to survive the horrors of the camps and prisons (Frankl, 1963; Henman, 2001). Humor has given people who were prisoners during war a sense of hope. It also established a bond among the prisoners (Frankl, 1963; Henman, 2001; Klein, 1998).

In his famous book, *Man's Search for Meaning,* Frankl (1963) discusses how even the smallest joke gave Holocaust prisoners such as himself a sense of hope. Humor helped give them something to look forward to each day. Frankl and a fellow prisoner would make up at least one amusing story each day. They joked with one another

about life after liberation. One of the stories from the camps is told by a person who was a child at the time of imprisonment. The individual recalls:

We mimicked top overseers, and I did impersonations about camp life and somebody did a little tap dance – different funny, crazy things. The overseers slipped into the barracks while we weren't looking, and instead of giving us a punishment they were laughing their heads off. I couldn't believe it. One day they were hitting us black and blue, and then they were laughing while we made fun of them. But, you see, in spite of all our agony and pain we never lost our ability to laugh at ourselves and our miserable situation. We had to make jokes to survive and save ourselves from deep depression (Klein, 1998, p. 149).

Henman (2001) views humor as a determinant of resilience and a method of recovery from the trauma of being a Vietnam POW. Henman did in-depth qualitative interviews with 12 Vietnam POWs who were imprisoned in the "Hanoi Hilton," one of the more notorious prisons. For these men, humor provided a means for building relationships. Humor also became a weapon for fighting back, a means of survival, and a way to remain resilient in the face of severe adversity.

Henman (2001) tells of one POW who realized the value of humor about 10 months after he was captured. The discovery of humor was a turning point for him. The event occurred while he was in solitary confinement. He was peeking through a hole in the wall and watching the guards. One of the guards must have asked for the time, but all he knew was that one guard had asked another guard a question. The POW saw the one guard hand his rifle to the other, then take off his bullet belt and his huge coat, and then reach into his pocket. After struggling with something in his pocket, he pulled out a Baby Ben clock. This struck the prisoner so funny, he started to laugh. He shared:

He didn't have a watch; he had a Baby Ben clock stuck in his pants pocket. And I'd been beaten pretty severely every day for most of a month, and I was just absolutely rolling on the floor. When this was over, I realized, "I thought I was going to die today; and all I did today was have a good laugh." And so it became apparent to [me] that humor was going to play a major role. (Henman, 2001, p. 86)

Several of the men in Henman's (2001) study told her that they felt humor was so important they would risk torture to tell a joke through the walls to a prisoner whom they felt needed cheering up.

Jeering and finding humor also seemed to be a covert way of fighting back or taking control in a situation in which there seemed to be no personal control. The prisoners established a process by which they could communicate with one another, even when it was dangerous to do so. In an interview for *USA Today* Representative Sam Johnson (R-Texas) talked about a "tap code" that was developed among the prisoners (Kiely, 2003). It was a simplified Morse code that was sometimes whispered from cell to cell, sometimes written in moistened cigarette ash with a bamboo twig on a piece of toilet paper, or even tapped on the wall. Some prisoners were able to tap out 30 words a minute. They also used a broom to sweep messages when they were forced to clean the prison yard. Using this form of communication, the prisoners could chat, share stories, and crack jokes. Retired General Robinson Risner remarked, "Humor was absolutely a necessity" (Kiely, 2003, p. 21).

If humor can promote survival among people undergoing this type of duress, it should be effective for any kind of stressful life event. Healthcare providers are often involved in one way or another with crisis situations. Understanding how humor can be beneficial during those times and how it can be incorporated and encouraged is important. It is also important to think about the following statement made by Captain Coffee to Paul McGhee

(2001): "Having some humor skills before being confronted by the adversity played a very important role." With that in mind, incorporating interventions to educate patients about humor might be a way of preventing PTSD when they are confronted with disasters and crises in their lives.

CASE STUDY

When Hurricane Katrina hit Biloxi, Mississippi, Mrs. Morrow was home alone. Her husband and adult son were stationed overseas, and her adult daughter was in Norfolk. It was just her and her dog at home. They evacuated, but a few days later Mrs. Morrow went back to her home, sneaking past street patrols. When her daughter finally reached her by phone she was relieved to find her mother and the dog survived the storm, but wondered how the house had faired. Mr. Morrow had just built a sunroom onto the house before he left. When the daughter inquired if all the windows were blown out, Mrs. Morrow humorously laughed and said, "Oh no, those windows were hurricane proof. They are lying on the lawn. The rest of the room is three houses down, though."

Questions

1. The type of humor used by Mrs. Morrow would most likely fall into which phase of disaster humor?

2. What purpose does disaster humor have?

3. What should disaster relief workers understand about using humor in disaster situations with individuals directly affected by the disaster?

Discussion

Mrs. Morrow's type of humor is most indicative of the honeymoon phase of disaster humor. During this phase of the disaster the survivor is happy to be alive. There is an element of denial concerning negative emotions or difficulties. The humor tends to laugh at the absurdity of the situation and there is little, if any, anger. This is demonstrated by her laughing at the fact that the windows, which her daughter seemed most concerned about, were fine, but the whole room was gone. The humor employed by survivors allows them to continue to cope with the situation. It helps express the feelings they are experiencing in a way that can help keep the stress of the disaster manageable.

Disaster humor can give disaster relief personnel a clue as to the phase of recovery the survivor is experiencing. Because this is a difficult and sensitive time for the worker and the survivor, it is important to realize that their appreciations for different types of humor will probably not be similar. The type of humor used by a disaster worker who is attempting to deal with "compassion fatigue" might be viewed as offensive or insensitive to the survivor, and vice versa.

SUMMARY

Even in disaster situations and crises, humor is an important coping mechanism. It has helped people survive terrorist attacks, natural disasters, and war imprisonment. Three factors needed for survivor recovery are relief from stress, talking about the experience, and passage of time. It is known that humor helps to relieve stress. Humor can also help set the stage for survivors to talk about their experiences.

Humor responses vary depending on the phase of disaster recovery the survivor is experiencing. Four phases of emotional recovery have been described: heroic, honeymoon, disillusionment, and reconstruction. Each of these phases supports different types of humor. Whereas the disaster survivor is attempting to make sense of the experience, the disaster relief workers are experiencing a sense of stress as they offer help and relief. The disaster worker and the survivor will see the same situation differently, so humor needs to be used judiciously. Also, the disaster relief worker may need to find an effective way to use humor away from those who are survivors.

Prisoners of war share that humor was a necessary part of emotional survival. Frankl, a survivor of the Holocaust and a psychologist, has written about his experience with humor as a means of giving prisoners a sense of hope. It is obvious that, even in crisis situations, humor is an important part of connecting, relieving stress, and surviving the negative experience.

EXAM QUESTIONS

CHAPTER 9
Questions 66-71

Note: Choose the one option that BEST answers each question.

66. Immediately after a tragedy, such as the attack on the World Trade Center, people respond with

    a. laughter to decrease tension.

    b. wonderment and humor.

    c. the inability to find humor.

    d. sarcastic humor aimed at the perpetrators.

67. The most common form of humor seen in disaster situations is

    a. incongruent-resolution humor.

    b. distancing humor.

    c. gallows humor.

    d. cartoons.

68. The emotional recovery phase that involves optimism is the

    a. heroic phase.

    b. honeymoon phase.

    c. disillusionment phase.

    d. reconstruction phase.

69. The type of disaster humor that reflects a "sense of community" is in the

    a. heroic phase.

    b. honeymoon phase.

    c. disillusionment phase.

    d. reconstruction phase.

70. Before using humor as a tool to assist a patient after a disaster, the first thing a healthcare provider should do is

    a. perform a humor assessment.

    b. assess the patient's phase of recovery.

    c. allow the patient to use humor first.

    d. make sure the patient has received some therapy.

71. Frankl stated that humor gave the prisoners of the Holocaust a sense of

    a. hope.

    b. pride.

    c. compassion.

    d. structure.

CHAPTER 10

HUMOR IN PSYCHIATRIC SETTINGS

CHAPTER OBJECTIVES

After completing this chapter, the reader will be able to discuss the effective use of humor in psychiatric settings.

LEARNING OBJECTIVES

After studying this chapter, the reader will be able to

1. identify the controversy that exists concerning the use of humor in psychiatric settings.

2. explain ways that humor can be used to diagnose a patient's psychological state.

3. discuss treatment options that include the use of humor in psychiatric settings.

4. recognize behaviors that indicate inappropriate responses to humor.

5. recount appropriate and inappropriate uses of humor in psychiatric settings.

6. discuss the use of humor by caregivers and the impact it has on patient care.

INTRODUCTION

The use of humor in psychiatric settings is a controversial issue. Although humor may be inappropriate with some psychiatric patients, with others it might be effective, appropriate, and helpful toward recovery. This chapter explores the use of humor in psychiatric settings. Topics include the reason for the controversy over the use of humor, ways to use humor for diagnosis and treatment, and psychiatric patient responses to humor. Appropriate and inappropriate responses and appropriate and inappropriate types of humor are discussed.

THE CONTROVERSY

The use of humor in therapy originally came from classical psychoanalysts (Robinson, 1991), who commonly followed the teachings of Freud. Interestingly, Freud was a pioneer in the area of humor and psychology. However, as Robinson (1991) notes, Freud's concentration on hostile wit rather than positive aspects of humor might be the cause of the modern controversy.

Mark Darby (1996), a psychiatric nurse, shares a story concerning the response of one of his coworkers when she witnessed his use of humor with a patient. The coworker pulled him aside and berated him for telling the patient a joke. She wanted to know, "How can we get patients to trust us if we laugh at them?" (p. 20). She continued to lecture him about appropriate etiquette with patients, which did not include room for even a good chuckle. The coworker was right in that trust is essential; however she was wrong in thinking that laughter and humor would destroy trust and rapport. There is a big difference between laughing with someone and laughing at someone. Humor, when used to laugh with someone, establishes a connection between the parties involved. Newirth (2006) notes that humor used in the analytic relationship can assist the patient's ability to symbolize unconscious experiences.

Some mental healthcare providers think that humor can be destructive to the therapeutic environment. This can be true if humor is used inappropriately. Others think that humor can be used to mask hostility and can be harmful if used incorrectly. Of course, inappropriate humor can be destructive to any therapeutic environment, not just the mental health environment. In contrast, humor used appropriately eases tension and can express warmth and caring.

Psychologist Joseph Newirth (2006) asserts that humor, like dreams, "facilitates the patient's development of the capacity to symbolize unconscious experience" (p. 580.) Whether initiated by the patient or the therapist, humor gives balance to the analytic relationship, merging the "unconscious experiences of the analyst and patient."

One study cited in Robinson (1991) found that patients with reactive depression (those who experience depression in response to a situation) responded to humor better than patients with psychotic depression. Patients with schizophrenic reactions showed increased ideation. Robinson (1991) mentions, "Although humor may facilitate the flow of free associations, it may block or arrest the patient's spontaneous stream of thought and may also confuse the patient as to whether the therapist is serious or 'only joking'" (p. 102).

Controversy exists concerning the use of humor with patients who have schizophrenia, especially paranoid schizophrenics who might think the care provider is laughing at them. In a qualitative study by Struthers (1999) on the use of humor by community psychiatric nurses, few of the nurses interviewed said they would not use humor with patients who demonstrated suspicious or paranoid behavior. A study by Gelkopf, Sigal, and Kramer

(1994) found that positive humor creates a positive atmosphere between patients and staff.

Interestingly, although controversy surrounds the use of humor in therapy, in a study by Haig (1988), almost 90% of therapists questioned said humor arose sometime during therapy, and 81% said they introduced jokes or humorous remarks during the therapy sessions. They reported they were most likely to use humor with patients who were anxious. The therapists also reported using humor with patients with obsessive disorders, personality disorders, and depression. They would occasionally introduce humor with psychotic patients.

As research continues on the use of humor in mental health care, it is hoped that the controversy concerning its use will decrease. A better question than "should humor be used in mental health settings?" is "how can humor be used effectively and with which type of patients is it most effective?"

HUMOR AS A DIAGNOSTIC TOOL

Although humor is not an effective measure of a psychological illness, it can be used as a means of assessing a patient's psychological state (Sultanoff, 2000).

Provine (2000a) discusses the inappropriate laughter that occurs in some subtypes of schizophrenia. He mentions that the *Diagnostic and Statistical Manual of Mental Disorders (DSM-IV)* lists silliness and laughter that are not related to content of speech as one of the symptoms for schizophrenia of the disorganized type. The behavior of inappropriate laughter could help lead to a specific diagnosis of this disorder (Provine, 2000a).

Humor might indicate an underlying issue that needs to be explored. Haig shares the story of a young woman whose sense of inferiority became apparent when she mentioned that she had not been born with a "bicycle pump." According to the story, a magician was away from home when his wife was due to give birth. He did not want to inform the audience or let the other performers know, so when the baby was born, he received a note saying, "The bicycle arrived safely, together with a bicycle pump." The young woman's father had wanted a son and she felt that she had not lived up to his expectations because she, unlike the magician's son, was born without a "bicycle pump" (p. 164). The inferiority she felt because she was not born a boy interfered with her attempts to relate to men. The sharing of this story led to her inferiority issue becoming the focal point of treatment (Haig, 1988).

According to Haig (1988),

Spontaneously arising humor and reactions to humor may indicate abnormalities in the underlying mood of the patient. The depressed individual may rarely find anything humorous…if he does, the humor is often "black" or tainted with irony… Laughter in the opening session often indicates discomfort or anxiety. Humor that arises suddenly with little apparent relevance to the topic being discussed may indicate denial, with repressed anxiety (p. 164).

There may be a number of reasons a person does not experience humor in their life. Some of these reasons can be excessive grief, chronic depression, inability to comprehend humor, or an inability to "let go" because of the need to be in constant control of his/her emotions (Goldin & Bordan, 1999). Some adult children of alcoholics might have a difficult time letting go and having fun because of the conditioning experienced as a child and the fear that the irresponsible behavior of their parents might afflict them if they are not in control (Woititz, 1983, cited in Goldin & Bordan, 1999). The inability to use and appreciate humor might be a clue that there are some issues that prevent the freedom of expression humor evokes.

Humor can be a measuring stick for assessing progression in therapy. While working with women who were diagnosed with posttraumatic stress disorder (PTSD), I found that humor was a measuring stick by which my two coleaders could monitor the group's progress. Humor was a tool that was often employed, and those women who were very depressed were less likely to laugh at humorous comments in the beginning of the session. Often, depression had lifted by the end of the session and smiles could be seen.

Sultanoff (2000) shares a story of a woman who felt that bad things happened to her because she was "stupid." He was able to assess her progress in therapy through a humorous statement concerning her sense of being stupid. When she responded to his comment with laughter, he assessed that she had made progress in therapy. If she had not responded with laughter, he would have diagnosed that she still had to work on that area of her belief system.

When working with a bereaved adult, a counselor can assess the patient's progress by his or her use of humor and laughter. At the beginning of an 8-week bereavement group, a 50-year-old gentleman shared details about his wife's death. As he started to share, he started to cry. The third week, the man told the group that he was diagnosed with bipolar disorder and was on medication. He rarely smiled, and he easily broke into tears. That 8-week session ended without much change in this man's affect. The counselors were concerned about him, and even though they knew he was under psychiatric care, they listened carefully for potential suicidal ideation. He requested to return for the next 8-week session. About halfway through the second session, the man began to smile and started kidding around with the counselors and some of the other members of the group. Although he still had bouts of depression, the depressive symptoms began to decrease. During the third 8-week session he attended, he started laughing and initiating funny stories. At this point, the counselors became more relaxed concerning his potential for suicidal ideation. The man's increased use of humor informed the counselors that the worst of the grief reaction had been worked through. The counselors felt that the gentleman's use of humor was appropriate and not being used to hide or suppress his feelings.

HUMOR AS TREATMENT

Humor "can promote insight by making repressed material conscious, resolving paradoxes, tempering aggression, and revealing new options" and it is a "socially acceptable form of sublimation" (Stuart & Sundeen, 1995, p. 44). That sentence sums up the role humor can play in treating mental illnesses. The rest of this section looks at the therapeutic value of humor as a treatment modality. Remember that humor is only one aspect of interactive care for mentally and emotionally distressed people.

Humor serves 14 functions within the nurse-patient relationship. Humor:

- establishes relationships
- decreases stress and tension
- promotes social closeness
- provides social control
- helps cognitive reframing
- reflects social change
- provides perspective
- expresses emotion
- facilitates learning
- reinforces self-concept
- voices social conflict
- assists with conflict avoidance
- facilitates enculturation
- instills hope.

(Stuart and Sundeen 1995)

Stuart and Sundeen (1995) also offer guidelines for the use of humor in the therapeutic milieu. They mention three main occasions when humor may be of therapeutic value, as well as the corresponding times when humor might be inappropriate (see Table10-1).

It is important to understand how humor can be used in a therapeutic relationship. First of all, humor builds relationships. It helps to establish rapport and can increase communication in a non-threatening manner. In order for therapy to be effective in the psychiatric arena, the healthcare provider must build a relationship with the patient. Humor can be used as a base on which to build a provider-patient relationship. The healthcare provider can use this base to respond to the patient in a way that facilitates growth (Sultanoff, 1992). However, if not used judiciously, humor can also hurt and destroy relationships.

Humor can also help catch a patient's attention and make messages more likely to be heard (Sultanoff, 1992). It can play a part in establishing

TABLE 10-1: GUIDELINES FOR THE USE OF HUMOR IN THE THERAPEUTIC MILIEU	
Therapeutic	**Inappropriate**
If the patient has mild to moderate levels of anxiety, functions as a tension reducer	If the patient has severe or panic levels of anxiety
When helping the patient cope more effectively, improving learning, putting life situations into perspective, and decreasing social distance. Understood by the patient for its therapeutic value	If it promotes maladaptive coping, masks feelings, increases social distance, or assists in avoidance of difficult situations
If it is consistent with social and cultural values of the patient, allows the patient to laugh at life, the human situation, or stressors	If it violates the patient's values, ridicules people, or belittles others
(Stuart & Sundeen, 1995, p. 43)	

and maintaining easier interaction between a patient and an analyst (Robinson, 1991). Sultanoff (1992) suggests that nurses and counselors use tools such as cartoons, anecdotes, jokes, puns, signs, and props to help illustrate the message they would like the patient to hear.

Humor can change how we feel. It is hard to experience humor and be depressed at the same time (Sultanoff, 1992). Here is a little experiment on how a smile can change your feelings:

- Make your face have a neutral expression – neither smiling nor frowning. Be aware of any feelings you might have.

- Make your facial expression a frown. Be aware of how you feel.

- Smile. Check out your feelings.

Many people who do this exercise find that they feel "lighter" when they smile. Was this the case for you? If it was, then you can understand the comment that it is hard to be depressed when you are experiencing humor. That does not mean that negative feelings will not return but, for the moment you may feel lighter. For psychiatric patients, depressed patients in particular, humor might offer a ray of hope that they could feel better, that they are not stuck in their depression.

Humor may also help reduce performance anxiety. For example, ask a patient to imagine a situation in which he or she experienced humor (Sultanoff, 1992). The patient can then learn to recall this situation when having an anxiety attack. This method helps reduce anxiety by substituting another feeling and by distracting the person from anxiety-producing thoughts.

How a person interprets events has a great impact on how that individual feels. The same set of events can elicit different feelings from different people. Humor can help change a person's thoughts about certain events, thereby changing his or her feelings (Sultanoff, 1992). Humor changes perceptions, and the change in perception alters feelings.

"That's the doctor who is treating me for paranoia. I don't trust him."

Note. From DansCartoons.com. Used with permission.

Personal Insight

While I was recovering from breast surgery, my husband and I were in California on a minivacation. I had developed an infection in the breast area that meant packing the wound with iodoform and changing dressings twice per day. It was a narrow, but deep wound. We had gone for a walk along a marsh area and suddenly my husband stopped and said, "I have to tell you something. It really bothers me to have to pack that wound, so I decided I needed to do something to personalize it. I thought about it and decided that packing the wound was like packing a flint lock musket, so I'm going to call it 'flint.' We both laughed and later we found that talking about "packing flint" made the dressing changes easier to deal with. Being able to laugh about it changed our perspective from something that was difficult to something that was bearable.

How people behave is linked to how they feel. As previously noted, humor can change the way a person feels; therefore it stands to reason that humor can change the way a person responds. Humor can help lighten a situation and encourage a person to try new things, take risks, and be open to possibilities (Sultanoff, 1992). When a care provider works with patients who have mental illnesses, a sign of improvement for the mentally ill is the willingness to take risks and try new ways of thinking and behaving.

Research shows that major depression alters immunity by decreasing natural killer (NK) cells (Bauer et al., 1995; Schleifer, Keller, Bartlett, Eckholdt, & Delaney, 1996;). NK cells assist in the prevention of cancer and viruses. Berk and Tan (1989, cited in Wooten, 1996) discovered that NK cells increase in response to laughter. In addition, studies indicate humor's potential for improving certain immune functions, such as immunoglobulin (Ig) A and IgG production. Humor that leads to laughter can help a person feel better physically. These changes all lead up to biochemical changes that can be beneficial for psychiatric patients.

As negative life events increase, people who use humor to cope report fewer mood disturbances than individuals who are less likely to use humor. Using humor to cope has been associated with more positive moods (Labott, Ahleman, Wolever, & Martin, 1990). Furthermore, laughter has positive effects on the cardiovascular, muscular, and skeletal systems.

In order to gain better understanding for potential interactions, Hugelshofer, Kwon, Reff, and Olson (2006) explored the use of humor for alteration in mood. They investigated the adaptive and maladaptive role of humor between attributional style and dysphoria. Attributional style refers to how people explain events that occur in their lives. They may see these events as stable or unstable, global (happening throughout one's life) or local (specific to a part of ones life), internal (within their control) or external (not within their control).

Through questionnaires that measured attributional style, humor styles, and depressive symptoms, they found that higher levels of affiliative humor (those who can easily joke around, tell amusing stories, laugh easily with others) and self-enhancing humor (ability to maintain a humorous outlook on life and use humor for coping) had fewer depressive symptoms. Hugleshofer et al. concluded that, although more research is needed, there is an indication that assisting people with depressive symptoms who exhibit negative attributional style in learning how to develop positive attributional humor might be an effective psychological intervention.

Humor has been used effectively in a number of counseling situations. These include group therapy, couple and family therapy, career and school counseling, as well as in analytic therapy (Goldin & Bordan, 1999). No matter what type of therapy is utilized, it is important to remember that humor can be detrimental as well as helpful. It must be judiciously used with an understanding of the positive as well as the negative power it might have. Enhancing or affiliative humor should be the only type of humor used. Clients who use self-effacing humor should be challenged because this type of humor is destructive to their self-esteem.

To use humor therapeutically, guidelines are important. Sultanoff (1994) believes it is important to look at

- the target of the humor (self, situations, or others);

- the environmental conditions in which humor is presented (with whom, at what time, and in what setting);

- and the specific person's receptivity to humor (what type of humor is the person comfortable with, what role does it play in his or her life, is the person able to laugh at himself or herself, and how does the person respond to the humor of others).

Pasquali (1995) talks about assessing timing (is this a good time for the client or are they in crisis mode); style (what type of humor is appropriate – joke telling, puns, slapstick, gallows, or funny stories and can they understand a particular style of humor); and context (similar to environmental conditions, this looks at the appropriateness of who, when, and what setting).

Goldin and Borden (1999) offer these reasons why humor may be ineffective:

- the counselor uses it to avoid the client's feelings.

- the client views it as not pertinent to his or her reason for counseling.

- it is used in a demeaning way.

- it is used too often and becomes boring.

- the timing is inappropriate.

Humor plays a part in a number of different types of therapy. Humor has been used effectively in behavior therapy, logotherapy, cognitive therapy, family and marital therapies, and group and milieu therapies (Haig, 1988).

HUMOR IN WORKING WITH THE CHRONICALLY MENTALLY ILL

Pasquali (1995) talks about the use of humor with chronically mentally ill (CMI) patients. Chronic mental illness can lead to defeatist feelings and behaviors in patients and healthcare providers. Mental illness can be a long-term problem with multiple challenges. The problems are not only emotional but also spiritual and social. Isolation of CMI patients is not uncommon. The chronicity of their problems can lead to frustration and feelings of hopelessness and helplessness for patients and healthcare providers. Incorporating humor therapy may help improve CMI patients' quality of life and provide a model that can help them function in the world (Pasquali, 1995).

Humor can be used successfully in the group setting, even with patients who have criminal pasts as well as psychiatric diagnoses. Minden (2002) conducted a qualitative study on the effects of a humor group on patients who were forensic psychiatric patients. These patients had committed such crimes as robbery, forgery, assault, arson, rape, incest, and murder. Their psychiatric disorders included anxiety disorder, impulse control disorder,

mood disorder, sexual disorders, and schizophrenia. Many of the patients had been or would be institutionalized for years. They tended to feel angry, helpless, and hopeless. Nursing students were used to facilitate the group with the support and guidance of their clinical instructor.

Rules for the humor group were established. Introductions were conducted at each group meeting due to patient turnover. The introductions set the tone by being conducted in a playful manner. Then, a call for jokes was made, which invited patients to share jokes that they knew as a way of sharing humor and preparing for more spontaneous humor. Humorous activities were also planned and sometimes involved patients and students working together. These activities included unique games, songs, dances, skits, or relays for which cooperation was emphasized. The sessions lasted an hour and often closed with talking about a funny group incident, another joke, or a goofy handshake.

After the experience, select members of the group were interviewed. The interviewees reported perceived benefits in their physical (46%), mental (100%), social (77%), and spiritual (46%) health (Minden, 2002). This group had deficits in their mental and social functioning. Minden (2002) notes that, in light of these deficits, "it is encouraging that so many found the group to have significant effects in these areas" (p. 81). One participant indicated that humor made the experience of a group appear less confrontational. "Humor made it easier to hear the feedback because I didn't feel like I was being attacked" (Minden, 2002, p. 82). This humor group intervention acknowledges that humor can be an effective addition to other types of therapy.

Gelkopf, Sigal, and Kramer (1994) studied the use of passive communal laughter to improve social support for a group of inpatients with chronic schizophrenia. The experiment was based on the theory that humor acts to relieve social fear and that laughing with others forms a more integrated psychological unit, increases group cohesiveness, establishes group membership, and relieves group tension. The researchers used humor videos with the experimental group and a combination of humor, romance, action, adventure, drama, and family films with the control group. The results of the study indicate that there was a perceived increase in support from the staff but not from fellow patients (Gelkopt et al., 1994). The researchers were unsure of the reason for the results; however, they noted that the introduction of laughter-stimulating videos appeared to change the social aspects between patients and staff. This did not occur with the control group. It would be interesting to see what would have happened if there was more interaction among the patients, as there had been in the study by Minden (2002).

Chato Stewart (2008), a cartoonist who has bipolar disorder, shares his humor and cartoons on the web with the hopes of helping others with mental illness find ways to laugh. He states:

> We know that even though we joke here and use humor to help deal with our disorders the fact is these mental health humor mug shots are serious issues! It is my hope that with the cartoons, I may in some way help educate and reduce stigma while tickling your funny bone once in a while.

One of his cartoons deals with the issue of peer support groups for the mentally ill.

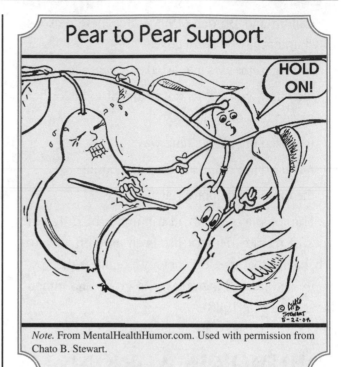

Note. From MentalHealthHumor.com. Used with permission from Chato B. Stewart.

APPROPRIATE HUMOR

Using humor in the psychiatric setting requires a more cautious approach than in the medical-surgical setting. Although the pointers offered in this section can apply to any patient experiencing the stress of illness, examples have been included to illustrate how they can be applied appropriately in the therapeutic environment for patients with mental disorders.

To determine the type of humor that might be appreciated and effective for a particular patient there are five areas that should be assessed:

1. attention span,
2. information access,
3. social cues processing,
4. decision making, and
5. focus.

(Darby, 1996)

Attention Span

Individuals with mental illness are likely to have short attention spans. These patients can concentrate on a single goal for a brief period of time and then quickly lose interest or divert to another thought or activity. Disease entities that seem to be characterized by the shortest attention spans are:

* *Major depression* – patients have difficulty concentrating and their thought processes are slowed.

* *Mania* – patients commonly suffer from excessive activity, loose association, and flight of ideas, making concentration difficult.

* *Schizophrenia* (depending on type and severity) – can cause people to have difficulty concentrating on what someone is saying to them; disorganized thinking may make following information difficult.

* *Attention deficit disorder* – For individuals with short attention spans, humor that has a short buildup would work best. The information presented needs to be delivered quickly. Spontaneous humor might be best for patients who demonstrate difficulty concentrating on information.

The following example illustrates the use of humor for someone with a short attention span:

A depressed patient with PTSD had been coming to group for a few weeks. She had demonstrated improved mood, but one week she came to the group feeling depressed. She stated that everyone was against her. Rather than responding in a way that indicated that the group members were not against her, the leader looked at her and said, "You're right, especially all of us here." She looked at the leader for a few seconds, and burst into laughter, acknowledging that she realized the all-or-nothing reaction she had was not valid.

Information Access

Individuals experiencing good mental health are usually able to process different pieces of information at once. As an example, a counselor notices that people are gathering outside a patient's room. One person

is crying, another is pacing, and another is standing and twisting a cloth in his hand. There is a sense of tension from the three people. The counselor may look at this scene and, through her visual, auditory, and kinesthetic senses, decide that something either is happening or has happened with the patient to cause the people outside the room to be upset. A patient suffering from a thought disorder would be unable to put this much information together. Rather, the patient may experience information overload, which may lead to a high-anxiety state.

When using humor with a patient who is mentally ill, it is important to assess how many and which channels of information work. The healthcare provider needs to know if the patient is better able to understand auditory, visual, or kinesthetic cues. Being observant and aware of how a patient learns information and responds to his environment should let the nurse or counselor know what avenue of humor the patient may be able to understand best. Patients who are auditory learners, and therefore learn best by hearing information, would understand spoken jokes or humorous statements best. Those patients who learn best visually would be more likely to understand written or visual humor. Patients who are kinesthetic might need someone to act out the joke or humorous information.

Social Cues Processing

Patients who are mentally ill sometimes have difficulty understanding social cues. Some patients may be able to understand abstract thought, but others are concrete thinkers. A concrete thinker, when asked what brought him to the hospital might say, "A taxi." Paranoid individuals are sure everyone is out to get them. For these people, implicit information needs to be made explicit. Darby (1996) demonstrates how to use humor with paranoid patients:

It was April Fool's week. Darby was working the night shift on an inpatient unit. A group of patients wanted to play as many practical jokes on the night shift as they possibly could. The night shift would respond in kind.

One of the patients was paranoid, and he watched what was going on with a rather tense look about him. Darby came up to the patient and asked, "How are things going, John?" The patient said, "I don't know what is going on, but I know that you guys are making fun of me."

At this point, Darby realized that he needed to defuse the patient's anxiety, so he took time to explain about April Fool's Day and attempted to teach him about the customs of that day. He took the implicit social cues and made them explicit through explanation.

After this explanation, John indicated he would like to be involved. He asked to have newspaper placed over his doorframe. When he woke up the next morning and saw his door covered with paper, he reacted as if he were completely surprised. He exhibited a joy much like a 6-year-old.

For someone who has difficulty perceiving social cues, the cues might need to be made explicit. Doing so in a way that does not ruin the punch line would allow an element of surprise. That element of surprise is what leads to something being humorous.

Decision Making

When trying to determine how a person understands and utilizes humor, it is important to assess the person's ability to make decisions. Patients who have difficulty making decisions have difficulty with too many variables. They can process information better with fewer variables. Understanding information or jokes is easier if they are presented in a simple manner. One way to assess a patient's ability to make decisions is to observe how he or she accomplishes tasks of daily living, such as deciding what to wear.

When using humor with patients who have difficulty making decisions, choose humor that requires fewer steps in understanding. Simple car-

toons require less processing of information than something as complex as a comedy film (Darby, 1996).

Focus

Some people can see the world in all of its beauty – the blueness of the sky, the flowers in bloom, the birds flying by. Others see the world through what Darby (1996) calls a "telephoto lens" (p. 85). A suicidal patient may be so focused on suicide as a means of relieving his emotional pain that he does not see the other options. Darby (1996) shares a story about a young man with obsessive-compulsive disorder. The patient was having difficulty controlling his compulsive need to count to 999 by threes. Using humor, Darby was able to help the patient take himself less seriously. Humor helped him to expand his focus and break his cycle. "If someone is focusing on a small portion of the world to the exclusion of everything else, humor should be directed toward expanding the focus of the individual" (Darby, 1996, p. 53).

There are some guidelines for healthcare providers to consider when introducing humor to patients who are CMI:

- Realize that clients may use humor to make an uncomfortable situation seem less fearful and anxiety-producing.

- Be aware of the amount of smiling and laughing the client engages in.

- Be open to silly and playful thoughts.

- Look for the absurdity in situations or recognize the incongruities.

- Laugh at incongruities in behaviors or situations, never at patient symptoms.

- Start by laughing at yourself.

- Look for opportunities to make others laugh.

- Look for the sunny side of life to develop your sense of humor. You do not have to tell jokes or be a comedian.

(Pasquali, 1995)

"It appears your HMO will only allow you 2 repressed memories, 1 childhood trauma, and 3 flashbacks per visit."

Note. From DansCartoons.com. Used with permission.

The guidelines presented above are intended for patients with mental health problems, but they can be used with other patients as well. Patients who are going through a crisis have a narrow focus, and may have difficulty making decisions, and may only be able to process one piece of information at a time. As important as it is to assess a mental health patient, it is just as important to assess any patient. Humor used inappropriately can be hurtful and damaging to the provider-patient relationship.

INAPPROPRIATE HUMOR IN THE MENTAL HEALTH SETTING

Because of the difficulties psychiatric patients may have in processing information and their potential for misinterpreting humor, it is important to be aware of when and what type of humor might be inappropriate. The controversy over using humor in therapy arose out of concern for its misuse; therefore, it is important to be aware of what would constitute misuse. Humor should not be used under the following circumstances:

- when the care provider uses it as a defense against his or her own anxieties;
- when the care provider uses it as a means of expressing his or her own hostility;
- when it is used as a means of ingratiating the care provider with the group;
- when there is confusion regarding whether the counselor is serious or joking;
- when it is used indiscriminately without considering the impact on the patient;
- when it belittles the patient;
- when it is used as a screen to avoid therapeutic intimacy;
- if the patient has severe or panic anxiety levels;
- if it encourages maladaptive coping responses, covers up feelings, increases social distancing, or helps the patient avoid dealing with difficult situations;
- when it violates someone's values.

(Robinson, 1991; Stuart & Sundeen, 1995)

EXAMPLES OF HUMOR USES IN MENTAL HEALTH

A 4-year-old boy shared jokes with his therapist as a way to diffuse the things he feared and to handle inner conflicts. The humor was mutually enjoyed. The young boy's teasing of the therapist seemed to represent a form of finding behavior that let him re-experience separation and reunion over and over (Haig, 1988).

A behavior therapist was working with a 21-year-old woman who was anxious because she was going to attend a banquet where she would meet her ex-boyfriend and his new girlfriend. The therapist employed systematic desensitization with the hope of decreasing her anxiety. Because there was not enough time for the patient to learn systematic relaxation, a humorous vision of her ex-boyfriend in leotards was used as she visualized herself at the banquet. This vision amused her and the evening went off well (Haig, 1988).

"A man with a repeated compulsion for checking the door at night was asked by his therapist to see how many times he could check the door in order to set a new record" (Haig, 1988, p. 146). The patient initially thought this was silly, but 3 days later the compulsion had disappeared.

Dealing with patients experiencing dementia can be challenging. Often, humor is one of the processes that can be affected because the ability to understand humor takes cognitive abilities. Patients with mild dementia become challenging because they are still able to recognize that they have a problem, and this can lead to depression. The following story told by Andrea Watson came from *Chicken Soup for the Nurse's Soul* edited by Canfield, Hansen, Mitchell-Autio & Thieman (2001). It was too touching and too revealing not to share.

Sadie, an 85-year-old woman, was in the hospital recovering from a heart attack. She had dementia, but could remember stories from her past that she loved to share. Her dementia was most apparent when she would ask questions about the recent past or couldn't find her way back to her bed from the restroom. On a few occasions, she tried getting into the bed of one of her four roommates, which caused an uproar. Sadie became sullen and quiet after these episodes.

One morning as Andrea started her rounds she noticed that Sadie was very sad. She seemed to want to share information but couldn't find the right words. After a few minutes Andrea realized Sadie had had an "accident" during the night and needed a good bath and a manicure. Andrea spent most of the morning soaking Sadie's hands in warm sudsy water. To ease Sadie's embarrassment, Andrea suggested she imagine she was spending the day being pampered at the beauty shop. They laughed together and played along until it was time to do her peri-care. As Andrea soaked her bottom,

Sadie became very quiet and her eyes "grew wide as saucers." Andrea asked if she were making Sadie uncomfortable in any way. Sadie looked at her and innocently said, "Honeychild, they've never done this to me at my beauty shop before!" Andrea bit her lip and told her "I certainly hope not," and then reminded her she was still in the hospital. They both laughed until they cried. That laughter seemed to be just what Sadie needed that morning to regain her dignity.

CASE STUDY

The following story is from the 1999 article by Goldin and Borden.

Betty, a 45-year-old married, unemployed, mother of two well-adjusted high school girls, sought counseling for depression. During the initial interview she told the counselor that although she had friends, was a good wife and mother, and felt as if she would be welcomed back to her former job, something was missing in her life. She intellectually appreciated her relationships, but she felt somehow unconnected to them emotionally. The counselor wished to develop rapport and attempted to communicate understanding, empathy, and interest in her concerns. The counselor also wished to assess her level of depression.

Betty: My family say they love and care for me. I appreciate it in here (pointing to her head), but I feel empty in my heart.

Counselor: Intellectually you know they are there for you. Somehow, it's just not convincingly getting through to you in here (points to heart).

Betty: And it makes me feel that maybe I'm really bad. Shouldn't I feel something?

Counselor: Like something's defective or just not good.

Betty: I know I'm not evil or something. I just want more and, honestly, they are all so needy. I sometimes think they are only there to get – I mean they're there, but they're really not there for me, or they're there as long as I keep giving, and that's not enough.

Counselor: Let me see if I have this straight. It seems as if they're present in your life, but not really there for you, and maybe even if they're there, it doesn't make it, it's not enough for you.

Betty: Yes, they're really selfish in many ways.

Counselor: You know, this reminds me of a counselor who saw someone who felt the way you do. She felt no one who was in her life was really there for her. The counselor meant to make her feel better, but it came out wrong. He said, "Well at least you always have yourself."

Betty: (laughing) But that's what it's like. They're not really there to give, and I don't feel I'm getting enough in my life.

Counselor: So, what do you think you need to get in order to feel that inside you were getting enough?

Questions

1. What was the purpose of using the story about the counselor and the other patient?

2. What information did the counselor gather about Betty's depression through the use of humor?

3. In what way was it effective?

Discussion

The story told by the counselor served two purposes. First it was a way of attempting to establish rapport and let the client know she was understood. It was also used to determine her level of depression. The fact that she laughed at the incongruity of the situation shared, informed the counselor of the depth of her depression. If she had not laughed the counselor may have felt that her depression level was deeper than it appeared. Because Betty was able to distance herself enough to see the humor in the remark, the counselor felt comfortable asking

her what she would need in order to feel that she was getting enough in her life. Because of the positive response to the remark, the counselor evaluated that the intervention was effective.

SUMMARY

Despite the controversy that exists concerning the use of humor in caring for patients who have mental illness, when used with sensitivity and knowledge, humor can be an adjunct to regular psychiatric care. This chapter has reviewed appropriate and inappropriate uses of humor in the therapeutic environment. In the psychiatric arena, as in other areas of health care, knowing when and how to use humor is essential.

Lessons for the chapter:

- Not everyone believes that humor is appropriate in the mental health setting.

- There is scientific research available that points to the efficacy of using humor in psychiatric or counseling situations.

- Humor can be a diagnostic tool.

  - Inability to use or appreciate humor might indicate abnormalities in underlying mood.

  - As psychiatric patients improve, humor is more easily accepted, and may begin to be used by the patients in a positive manner.

- Humor can be an adjunct to the treatment plan.

  - It can bring repressed material to the surface.

  - It helps establish a bond between patient and practitioner.

  - Stuart and Sundeen list 14 different functions humor has in the practitioner-patient relationship.

- There are three main functions of humor in the therapeutic relationship

  - It builds a practitioner-patient relationship.

  - It catches the patient's attention with the hope that messages will be heard; promotes insight.

  - It changes how people feel.

- Humor can help reduce performance anxiety.

- Humor can change perspective and perception of self or events.

- People who use humor report less mood disturbances.

- Guidelines for using humor:

  - Assess timing.

  - Assess type of humor and avoid hurtful humor.

  - Assess respectability.

  - Assess which channels of information work for that patient.

    o   Auditory

    o   Visual

    o   Kinesthetic

- Humor can be used effectively with patients considered seriously mentally ill.

  - It must be used carefully and the practitioner must be knowledgeable in therapeutic humor.

  - When used with patients having short attention spans, humor should delivered quickly – no long buildup or stories because they will lose interest.

- Times when humor should not be used to include

  - when it is being used for the practitioner's comfort, not the patient's,

  - when is belittles or is obscure,

  - if the patient is a severe or panic level,

  - when it is maladaptive for the patient.

EXAM QUESTIONS

CHAPTER 10
Questions 72-79

Note: Choose the one option that BEST answers each question.

72. There are many reasons for the controversy over the use of humor in the psychiatric setting. Robinson (1991) attributes the cause of this modern controversy to

    a. a psychiatrist's own discomfort with the use of humor.
    b. the stereotypical belief that psychiatric patients are unable to appreciate humor.
    c. Freud's concentration on hostile wit rather than the positive aspects of humor.
    d. the proven lack of therapeutic effect humor has in this setting.

73. Inappropriate laughter occurs in the diagnosis of

    a. borderline personality disorder.
    b. bipolar, depressive type.
    c. schizophrenia, disorganized type.
    d. clinical depression.

74. Humor can be used in a diagnostic manner with psychiatric patients to

    a. diagnose the specific illness.
    b. assess patient's progress.
    c. diagnose the disorder without further testing.
    d. label the disease process according to the *Diagnostic and Statistical Manual of Mental Disorders,* 4th Ed.

75. One of the most important uses of humor by the practitioner in the psychiatric setting is as a

    a. means for the patient to poke fun at his illness.
    b. method of promoting insight.
    c. way of provoking laughter.
    d. means of facing reality.

76. According to Stuart and Sundeen (1995), the use of humor in a therapeutic milieu is considered appropriate when it

    a. ridicules people and violates their values.
    b. puts life situations into perspective.
    c. promotes social distance from one another.
    d. assists in avoiding difficult situations.

77. When determining which type of humor to use with a patient, Darby suggests assessing five areas, including

    a. attention span.
    b. favorite sitcom.
    c. laugh triggers.
    d. affect.

78. When planning humor interventions, anticipate a short attention span in patients with

    a. obsessive-compulsive disorder.
    b. narcissistic personality disorder.
    c. somatoform disorder.
    d. mania.

79. Humor, when used by the mental health worker, is inappropriate when

    a. puns are used.

    b. humorous props are used.

    c. it belittles the patient.

    d. it attempts to change others' perspectives.

CHAPTER 11

HUMOR AND LEARNING

CHAPTER OBJECTIVES

After completing this chapter, the reader will be able to discuss the ways in which humor can be used in educational situations.

LEARNING OBJECTIVES

After studying this chapter, the reader will be able to

1. describe the effects of humor on learning.

2. demonstrate an understanding of learning theories.

3. describe the effects of aging on learning.

4. discuss ways in which humor can effectively be incorporated into healthcare education.

5. differentiate between positive and negative types of humor in learning.

INTRODUCTION

People rarely succeed unless they have fun in what they are doing.

– Dale Carnegie

For many people, the times when they have most enjoyed learning – and often the times when they have learned the most – are when instructors have interjected humor or used exercises to make learning fun. There was a time when people commonly believed that teachers needed to be very serious because learning was considered a serious business. However, we now know that having fun when you learn helps increase the ability to learn and retain information. This chapter discusses theories about how people learn, presents research on the importance of humor in education, talks about the use of humor in healthcare and patient education, and offers a few examples.

WHY HUMOR?

When trying to learn new material, tension can be a hindrance. When people are upset, anxious, or concerned about something, learning new material can be very difficult. They may find it is easier to focus on the problem rather than the solution. In order for a student to be able to concentrate and learn new information, it is important for the teacher to promote some form of relaxation. For example, if a nurse is trying to teach a patient with diabetes, and the patient has a fear of needles, the patient may not hear anything the nurse says. It has been found that humor in the classroom assists in increasing motivation, reducing tension, and aiding in instruction (Flowers, 2001). If this can happen in the classroom, it can likely happen during patient education as well, whether that education is one-on-one or in a group.

Research also shows increased retention of information when humor is used in teaching (Kaplan & Pascoe, 1977; Lamp, 1992). One strategy that has been used to educate postpartum parents about the reality of adapting to a new baby is "Fredricka, A New Mother's Worst Nightmare" (Lamp, 1992).

Fredricka visits postpartum patients on their day of discharge dressed in a manner that humorously depicts the disheveled, fatigued new mother. She appears in a tousled wig with curlers, a bathrobe, slippers, dark circles under her eyes, a laundry basket filled with linen, and a toddler-sized doll attached and clinging at knee-level to the robe. She discusses such issues as fatigue, role transition, sibling rivalry, self-image, involution, breast changes, sexual intercourse, the hormonal influences on emotions, and nutrition.

Patients were quite attentive to this humorous approach. Lamp (1992) noted that the information taught was retained and transcended cultural, developmental, socioeconomic, and educational boundaries.

Humor also seems to increase the ability to think creatively. A study by Isen, Daubman, and Nowicki (1987) demonstrated that people exposed to a few minutes of a comedy film performed better on a problem-solving task than a control group that was not exposed to comedy. Humor may have a

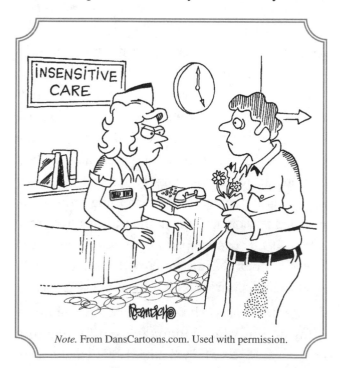

Note. From DansCartoons.com. Used with permission.

positive effect on people, causing them to improve their problem-solving performance. Humor may also play a role in assisting students to make new discoveries and better, more creative decisions.

Robinson (1991) states, "the concepts of creativity and change are closely related to each other as well as to humor and learning" (p. 119). The goal of education is to facilitate change and learning. Creativity, which includes the use of humor, can lead to change. For the educator, it can lead to a change in the methods used for presentation. For the learner, it can assist in the process of understanding and moving toward change.

HUMOR'S ROLE IN LEARNING

In addition to reducing tension, humor helps make concepts that might be difficult easier to understand and retain (Bartlett, 2003). As noted by *Humor Project* creator Joel Goodman (Millbower, 2010), humor helps the learner go from "HaHa" to "aHa!" Humor captures the learner's attention and holds that attention, increasing the person's motivation and interest in learning. If the person is interested in learning, the information is more likely to be retained. However, this theory is controversial.

A number of studies did not show improved retention with the use of humor (Whisonant, 1998). Most of these studies were done in one day, however this finding held true even in studies in which posttests were given 1 week later. Interestingly, a study by Kaplan and Pascoe (1977) showed that, although the participants had no immediate effects on retention, there was significantly more effective retention of information for those participants who viewed humorous items than those who viewed nonhumorous items when they took a post-test 6 weeks later.

Studies have examined the effect of humor when related to patient teaching. A study reported by Delp and Jones in 1996 (cited in Schrecengost,

2001) explored the effects of cartoons on patient comprehension of and compliance with wound care instructions. The experimental group received instructions that contained cartoons, and the control group received instructions without cartoons. The patients in the experimental group were more likely to have read the discharge instructions, more likely to answer all the wound care questions correctly, and more compliant with wound care. This study indicates that cartoon illustrations can be an effective teaching tool and may improve patient compliance with wound care instructions.

Schrecengost (2001) studied the effects of humor on postoperative teaching among 50 patients who were scheduled to undergo coronary artery bypass graft or valve surgery. All the patients were presented with a patient-teaching booklet. The experimental group received a booklet with cartoons representing three postoperative exercises. The control group's booklet did not contain cartoons. Both booklets contained the same information. The results of this study indicate that both groups had improved knowledge. Although there was no statistically significant difference in knowledge, the experimental group did slightly better on the post-test.

Humor is important in academic learning. It helps to increase students' self-esteem, sense of empowerment, and confidence in being able to learn the material. Humor in the classroom also helps to reduce tension, stress, anxiety, and boredom while helping to increase problem solving and promote creativity. Perhaps most importantly, inclusion of humor in classroom instruction has been shown to increase retention of the material presented. (Berk, 2002, Martin, 2007).

LEARNING THEORIES

Incorporating effective, appropriate humor into teaching is easier when the educator understands how people learn. This section presents information that may be useful in assisting nurses to comfortably add humor to their patient-teaching styles. Malouf (2003) states that teaching is a skill. The best way to develop a skill is to understand the underlying process and to practice. To understand how to be an effective teacher, it is important to understand theories of how people learn.

Overview of Learning Theories

How people gather, process, remember, and use information has captured the interest of philosophers, psychologists, and various other individuals for years. As a result, there are many learning theories. A few of these theories are discussed here.

Bower and Hilgard (1981) note that there are basically two opposing positions on how knowledge is acquired: *empiricism* and *rationalism.* Those who subscribe to the empiricism theory believe that all knowledge evolves through sensory experience. Rationalism, in contrast, involves the belief that reason is the main source of knowledge. It is reason, rather than data obtained through sensory experience, that is the basis of knowledge.

Descartes, Kant, and other rationalists believed that relationships between basic sense points were as primary and psychologically intense as the sense points themselves. As an example, when we listen to music, we do not hear just the tones, but coherent melody (Bower and Hilgard, 1981). When we hear a joke, it is the recognition of the incongruity that allows us to "get it."

Empiricism and rationalism provide the background for more modern learning theories. Pavlov and Skinner, who subscribed to the empiricism theory, are two of the names most commonly connected with the *stimulus response theory.* Many individuals are familiar with the story of Pavlov and his dog, in which ringing a bell caused the dog to salivate even when no food was presented. According to this theory, learning takes place when a stimulus represents an event. The ringing of the bell represents the presentation of food. Eventually, the animal or person responds in a predictable manner (salivation) without the presentation of the reward (food).

Skinner's theory of learning also deals with behavior responses. He believed that learned behavior affected subsequent behaviors (Dworetzky & Davis, 1989; Hergenhahn, 1990; Murphy, 1978). This theory is known as operant conditioning. For example, if a young child played with a television set and was told "no" often enough, the child would learn that the television was not something with which to play. Or, in the field of humor, if a child is told that being silly is not proper behavior, he or she learns that actions others might find silly, but he or she finds enjoyable, are not okay. Positive reinforcement of behavior is more likely to result in repetition of that behavior (Hergenhahn, 1990).

Arguments against Skinner's theory focus on the concept of cause and effect. However, for many years, Skinner's principles have been used in schools. Students are rewarded (behavior reinforcement) for doing well in class by such methods as positive affirmations, high grades, and praise. Students begin to recognize that parcels of knowledge can be applied to other situations. Although more information on how learning takes place has become available over the years, some of the operant conditioning principles are still applicable today.

One part of operant conditioning that might be a concern in educating others is that children are taught that education is serious – that clowning around when you are supposed to be learning is not appropriate. This conditioning can have a negative effect because the child may not recognize that use of humor and play does not mean that the teacher of the material should not be taken seriously. Research has demonstrated that some material is retained more effectively if humor and play are used in teaching (Berk, 2002; Humor Project, Inc., n.d.; Kaplan & Pascoe, 1977). Learning may be

serious business, but that does not mean it cannot be fun.

Learning also takes place through observation of the behaviors of others. Using research on the influences of social behavior, Albert Bandura pioneered the *social learning theory* (Murphy, 1978). Bandura (1997) notes that behavior is influenced by what people think, feel, and believe. Behavior is the result of the interplay between the individual's personal self-system and external sources of influence (Hergenhahn, 1990; Pajares, 1997).

Social cognitive theory assumes:

- reciprocal interactions exist between individuals, behaviors, and the environment;

- learning can be enactive and vicarious;

- maturation and experience increase a person's knowledge;

- there is a distinction between learning and performance.

The term *reciprocal interactions* refers to interacting environmental variables, behaviors, and personal factors, such as the person's analysis of the situation (Hergenhahn, 1990; Schunk, 1991). Each individual brings to a situation his past personal experiences in the context of the present situation. How events turn out in the present situation will, in turn, help determine the response in the next situation (Hergenhahn, 1990).

Enactive learning takes place when a person learns from his or her own actions. *Vicarious learning* takes place by listening to or observing others or by reading. For example, a nurse can teach a patient how to perform a procedure such as insulin injection by demonstrating the procedure and then having the patient demonstrate the procedure back to the nurse. Or, the patient can read about preventive measures and evaluate the results of their learning by discussing what they understood and receiving feedback from the nurse and others.

Another assumption of social cognitive theory is the distinction made between learning and performance of previously learned behaviors (Schunk, 1991). In other words, just because one knows how to do something, doesn't mean he will actually do it. Social cognitive theory outlines three types of knowledge: declarative, procedural, and conditional. *Declarative* knowledge includes facts, scripts, and organized passages. Concepts, rules, and algorithms are examples of *procedural* knowledge. *Conditional* knowledge refers to "knowing when to employ forms of declarative and procedural knowledge and why it is important to do so" (Schunk, 1991, p. 104).

Much of the time, declarative, procedural, and conditional knowledge interact (Schunk, 1991). For example, during a lecture, participants think about what's being presented (environment influences cognition). Participants who do not understand ask questions about the presentation (conditions influence behavior). The presenter responds to the question (behavior influences environment). The presenter asks the participants to engage in an experiential experience (environment influences cognitions, which influence behavior). The participants enjoy the activity and request more time to experience the results, and the presenter grants the time (cognitions influence behavior, which influences environment).

Modeling is a social theory concept that refers to behavioral, cognitive, and affective changes that occur after observing one or more models (Schunk, 1991). Observing another person modeling a behavior can strengthen or weaken a previously learned behavior. An example of observational learning is if someone at a humor program notices others around him being playful and, although it may be out of character, tries the playful behaviors to see how it feels.

Modeling can also take place when a nurse laughs at herself for a mistake that she made, such as mispronouncing a word. This response can also

help to reduce stress. Stress relief can be further demonstrated by asking the patient to join in a laughing exercise. If the nurse starts to laugh, the patient will most likely follow the example because laughter tends to be contagious. After the laughter exercise, the nurse can ask the patient to describe what he or she felt, and the nurse can build on that sharing to talk about the ways laughter and humor can help decrease tension and change the perspective of a situation.

Modeling involves attention, retention, production, and motivation (Hergenhahn, 1990; Kearsley, 1997; Schunk, 1991). Attention refers to things a person notices in his or her environment (Berk, 2002). People are most likely to attend to things or events they find valuable or interesting (Hergenhahn, 1990; Kearsley, 1997).

Retention is the storage of information and includes the ability to recall what has been coded, cognitively organized, symbolically rehearsed, or rehearsed through movement or physical manipulation (Hergenhahn, 1990; Kearsley, 1997; Schunk, 1991). Colorful cartoons, humorous songs, and specific movements tend to hold people's attention and increase retention (Berk, 2002).

Production refers to demonstrating or performing the modeled event. This process occurs when patients or students demonstrate that they have learned a skill or information that has been modeled. By practicing the skills learned and receiving feedback, learners can refine their knowledge and perform skills more accurately (Schunk, 1991).

Motivation may occur from within or it may be external (Huitt, 2001). According to social learning theory, reinforcement, either direct (experiencing their own consequences for behavior) or vicarious (seeing how others have consequences applied to their behaviors) provides the motivation for action (Hergenhahn, 1990; Huitt, 2001). Individuals are more likely to be motivated to adopt behaviors if the behaviors result in outcomes they value (Hergenhahn, 1990; Kearsley, 1997). Humor is a positive means of reinforcing the information and may increase the motivation to continue learning.

Social learning theory recognizes that individuals develop performance standards by which they evaluate their own behavior. They maintain this behavior through self-regulation (Hergenhahn, 1990). *Self-efficacy* is an important variable in determining self-regulatory behavior (Hergenhahn, 1990). According to Bandura (1997), self-efficacy is a belief in one's ability to organize and implement actions necessary to reach designated performance levels. Individuals who do not see that they have the ability to succeed can be encouraged and supported by others to reach their goals and to make the effort to succeed.

According to Kearsley (1997), the main principles of Bandura's social learning theory are as follows:

- Organizing and rehearsing modeled behavior symbolically and then performing it overtly will result in the highest level of observational learning. By coding modeled behavior into images, labels, or words, better retention will occur than with observation alone.

- Modeled behavior is more likely to be adopted if there is perceived value.

- A modeled behavior is more likely to be adopted if the model has admired status and the behavior has functional value.

Adult Learning Theories

Today, it is recognized that adults learn differently from children. Until the 20th century, however, the theoretical framework for all education was *pedagogy* (Knowles, 1978). The literal meaning of the term pedagogy is the art and science of teaching children. After World War I, there emerged an increasing notion that adults had unique characteristics as learners (Knowles, 1978). It was recognized that adults enter the learning process with more prior knowledge than children. Adults display increased variability due to experiences, culture, prior learning, and other influences on their knowledge. They also display less plasticity, or moldability, than children (Long, 1990).

Malcolm Knowles, a recognized expert in adult education, uses the term *andragogy* to describe his model of adult learning (Goodboe, 1995; Merriam & Brockett, 1997). Knowles (1978) lists four main assumptions of andragogy:

1. Adults prefer to be self-directed.

2. Adults bring unique life experiences with them to the learning situation. These experiences can be used as a resource for learning.

3. Adults' willingness to learn is usually linked to what adults consider relevant. It is believed that adults will learn faster and with more lasting results if the material is significant to them and to their present lives (Vella, 1994).

4. Adults' orientation to learning is problem-centered (Knowles, 1978). Adults tend to seek out learning because they have use for the knowledge or the skill being taught. "Learning is a means to an end, not an end in itself" (Zemke & Zemke, 1984, p. 1).

A number of characteristics specific to adult learners have emerged (Malouf, 2003; Merriam & Brockett, 1997; Taylor & Burgess, 1995). Nurses need to understand how to present material that will meet the expectations and needs of these learners. Table 11-1 depicts adult learner characteristics and points to keep in mind when designing educational programs.

Most adults are self-directed learners. Self-directed learners know what they want to learn and are willing to accept responsibility for discovering the information and resources necessary to meet their needs or desires related to acquisition of that knowledge (Brookfield, 1986; Knowles, 1978). Some researchers define *self-directedness* as a learner's ability to independently plan, conduct, and evaluate his or her own learning experience (Brookfield, 1986). Brookfield (1986) cautions that using the term self-directed might indicate that the

TABLE 11-1: SUMMARY OF ADULT LEARNER CHARACTERISTICS		
Characteristics	**Potential Barriers**	**Approaches**
Many prior experiences	Prior experiences might match present knowledge, as can be seen in changes in childrearing practices over the years.	Utilize what learners already know and build on it.
Set habits and strongly established expectations	Habits are easier to make than to break. Learning requires change, and change may be resisted.	In order to facilitate change, make learners feel safe. Humor results in a relaxed atmosphere that can encourage learning.
Many preoccupations	Maintaining attention may be a challenge.	To keep and hold attention, use visuals. Have learners participate in learning. Make it fun.
Attitudes often firmly established	Learning new material, especially if it requires a change in lifestyle, can be difficult.	Make learners understand why new behaviors would be better than the old in order to promote change.
Specific purpose for learning	Learners may feel as if the information to be learned does not apply to them.	Show learners that the learning will satisfy their needs, solve a problem, and be used immediately.

(Knowles, 1978)

person is wholly in control of the learning process. It is important to remember that no individual can undertake the process of learning or education without some external sources or stimuli.

Studies undertaken by Brookfield and others indicate some need for careful utilization of terminology when viewing self-directedness in the light of independent or dependent learning (Brookfield, 1986). Studies of individuals from different cultures indicate that people who score high on self-directedness may prefer dependent learning techniques.

Brookfield (1986) states, "Successful self-directed learners appear to be highly aware of context in the sense of placing their learning within a social setting in which advice, information, and the skill modeling provided by other learners are crucial conditions for self-directed learning" (p. 44).

Adult learners are motivated to learn in order to cope with specific life-changing events, such as marriage, a new job, a promotion, illness, losing a job, or divorce. As the stress of such life changes

accumulates, the motivation to cope with these changes through learning increases. When adults are convinced that change is inevitable, they will participate in any learning that appears to be able to help them cope with the transition (Long, 1990; Zemke & Zemke, 1984).

Some adults have personal growth motives, and participate in learning to become more informed individuals. Others choose learning experiences to meet new and interesting people. Skill acquisition that results in a way to spend spare time more enjoyably, such as skiing or scuba diving, may be the motivation for learning. In other words, there are many motivators for adult learning. These motivators can result in self-directed learning. Finding out what motives stimulate patients to learn can assist in designing patient-education programs (Long, 1990).

The term *motivation* is used by psychologists to describe processes that stimulate behavior and give purpose or direction to the behavior. Functions seen as necessary in learning, such as concentration, attention, effort, perseverance, and initiative, can be strongly influenced by a person's internal or external environment. Wlodkowski (1990) states that these influences make motivation unstable. According to Wlodkowski (1990), factors that help maintain motivation include feeling successful, viewing efforts as worthwhile or valuable, and experiencing pleasure in the learning. Humor can be a motivator in learning (Hudson, 2001; Lomax & Moosavi, 2002).

Not all adult learners are self-directed (Grow, 1996). Individuals come to the learning environment at different stages of life development. Students who are accustomed to directive learning feel uncomfortable in a self-directed learning environment. These individuals want and expect the facilitator to be in control of the learning environment. They also expect lecture presentations that allow them to listen, practice, and receive immediate correction. Other learners may enter the learning environment with some desire to be in control of their own learning but need and seek guidance in methods of acquiring information. As students become more self-directed, they tend to desire fewer teacher-directed activities.

Diversity is a key word when thinking about adult learners. Because adults bring to the learning environment different physiological, psychological, and sociological experiences, speaking of an "adult learner" as if there is a generic adult is erroneous (Long, 1990). Adult learners can range in age from 20 to 90 or more. Learning abilities, prior knowledge, physiological issues, and many other factors are involved in determining how and what an adult learner may learn.

Effects of Aging on Learning

As educators, nurses must also consider the needs of older adults. Who is considered an older adult learner? Do older adults continue to be involved with learning? What effects do memory and brain changes have on older adult learning? In what ways do older adults learn differently from younger adults? Some authors refer to individuals ages 50 and older as older adults (Kidd, 1990; Lumsden, 1987-1988). The Elderhostel program, a program designed for older adults, is available for individuals older than age 55 (Elderhostel, n.d.). Kleiman (1995) refers to individuals ages 55 to 65 as young old.

As adults age, their interest in education changes and their ability to learn changes. However, change does not necessarily mean a decrease in ability.

Physiological changes that occur with aging can affect the speed of information gathering. Many adults in their 40s begin to develop presbyopia, a condition that requires bifocals, or the use of magnifying devices. Adjustment to these visual assistive devices can increase assimilation difficulty, especially if learning involves the use of print and projected media, requiring the learner to shift fields of vision from 18 inches to 20 feet and then back again (Long, 1990).

Another normal aspect of aging that can affect the learning ability of an individual is impaired hearing. In fact, older learners express concerns about reduced hearing abilities more often than they do about visual problems. One problem related to impaired hearing is a lack of awareness on the part of the learner. *Patient: I have a new hearing aid. Nurse: What kind is it? Patient: One o'clock* (Buxman, 2000, p. 32). Hearing deficits related to age commonly occur insidiously, so the individual may not be aware of the problem. Presbycusis, a hearing defect that involves inability to hear high-pitched sounds, leads to misinterpretation of words because certain sounds are harder to discern (Long, 1990).

As adults age, their subcutaneous fat decreases and the body's ability to maintain heat changes. Therefore, the room should be a comfortable temperature for the participants. Most older adults prefer a room that is on the warm side.

Another age-related concern is energy expenditure. For some older adults, age brings with it a decrease in energy level. This factor can lead to increased fatigue that results in decreased attention levels. Long (1990) notes that teachers need to be sensitive to older learners' physical expenditure needs in order to keep them engaged in the learning process. Humor works as a stimulator and, according to Berk (2002), it can "increase the students' mental and physical pain tolerance for sitting through" the class or lesson (p. 60).

Beliefs about cognitive issues in aging can lead to educator bias. Unfortunately, some individuals believe that the ability to learn decreases with age. Although studies indicate that there is some slowing of the cognitive processes with aging (Ferraro, 1997; Knight, 1996), Ferraro (1997) notes that, with normal aging, decline in problem solving was found only among those in their 70s. Knight (1996) discusses that the use of working memory declines with age. Age-related changes could decrease the pace and increase the effort of new learning as well as affect language comprehension. This does not mean, however, that the older adult cannot learn new information; it just means that the presentation of the information may need to be adjusted to meet the needs of older adults. Humorous or playful interactions that remind older learners of their former experiences and tap into their former knowledge may be beneficial in the learning process. Remember, however, that the comprehension of the punch line in jokes may decrease with age (Kingsley, 2003). As the frontal lobe in the brain deteriorates with aging, mental flexibility, the ability to perform abstract reasoning, and working memory may be affected, which may be the reasons for decreased humor comprehension.

Studies indicate that the tendency to attend formal education declines with age. However, informal learning projects seem to increase with age. It has been suggested that perhaps "at some point during the adult years, there occurs a shift from a preference for institutionally sponsored educational activities to a preference for self-initiated, self-planned, self-directed learning" (Lumsden, 1987-88, p. 11).

McCullough-Brabson (1995), a music educator who teaches for Elderhostel, discusses her experience with older adult learners. While doing an informal survey, she discovered reasons people attended Elderhostel programs. These reasons included the excitement of the learning experience, an economical way to get good food, comfortable lodging, well-done programs, a stimulating vacation, and a desire and interest in learning new things. She shares her ingredients for success with teaching the older adult. She notes that the facilitator needs to know the subject material very well. Organization and preparedness are important. Older adults want an "organizational road map" in the form of a detailed syllabus so that they know the objectives and the plan for each day and class session. She suggests using various methods, such as videos, hands-on experience, and field trips, to illustrate major points. Enthusiasm, animation, and a sense of humor are important characteristics of a good facilitator. It is also important for the facilitator to allow time for comments and questions but to control the class if someone tends to monopolize the session. The need for awareness of the physical needs of older adults is stressed. Facilitators should use visual aids that are large and easy to read. When the facilitator is designing handouts or overheads, it is important to remember that dark words on a light background are easiest to read.

ADDING HUMOR TO HEALTHCARE EDUCATION

Now that we have some understanding of how scientists believe people learn, let us explore what can be done to increase learning through humor. The use of humor must be tasteful, not hurtful, and it must relate to the topic in order to be meaningful for the adult learner. Whether you are teaching to individuals, groups, or students, incorporating humor can enhance your lessons and improve attention and retention.

Some people are uncomfortable about adding humor to their teaching material because they cannot tell jokes. The ability to tell jokes is not necessary for the addition of humor in an educational session. Using visual aids helps increase understanding, so using cartoons or cartoon-type figures might be one way of adding humor that does not involve telling jokes. The idea of using humor is not to put on a show but to find a way that is comfortable for you to interject humor where appropriate (Hudson, 2001).

Another aspect of using humor is being open to it. Be alert to ways of presenting information without putting other people down. If possible, make yourself the object of the humor. The trick to education is for teachers to make sure they do not shut off humor as a tool. A funny presenter does not have to tell funny stories; he or she just needs to connect with common truths that will bring out the humor response (Masie, 2003).

The following example illustrates how to use humor to teach patients about proper alignment following hip surgery:

> Share with the patient that, when cutting up a chicken, to dislocate and remove the thigh at the hip, you bring the chicken's thigh toward its body and rotate it inward and toward the center, causing the hip to pop. If the patient does not want to be a chicken, he or she needs to be sure to not repeat that action.

If you make a mistake or use the wrong words when explaining something, make light of the situation in some way. Making a comment such as, "my mouth runs faster than my brain" can help to demonstrate in a humorous manner that mistakes happen and are just a part of life. If the nurse can laugh at herself, hopefully the patient will recognize

that everyone makes mistakes and, therefore, will not be as anxious about learning new material. Humor is viewed as a way to humanize the relationship between student and teacher (Lawson, 2001).

When providing patient teaching, the nurse needs to be alert to subtle uses of humor by the patient. This humor can provide clues to the patient's anxieties and hopes (Lawson, 2001). A patient's humor usage can also provide clues about financial concerns, family pressures, and fear of failing.

SUGGESTIONS FOR THE HEALTHCARE EDUCATOR

For those who teach healthcare providers or continuing education for healthcare personnel, here are a few suggestions for ways to add humor into your educational process. If your job is to design math quizzes for nurses, add a few humorous questions. The following are suggestions by Sue Moore (2002) taken from the Web site www.allnurses.com.

- You are assisting a primary nurse with charcoal administration down an orogastric tube. The room measures 8 ft by 12 ft. The patient starts to retch before the tube is pulled. Knowing that charcoal can spew out of a tube in a 5-ft radius (even with a thumb over the opening) and the stretcher is 2 ft wide, how many feet per second must you back up to get less charcoal on you than the primary nurse?

- You were assigned two large treatment rooms and the gynecologic room. By the end of the day, you have cared for ten patients. Four patients were females older than age 80, all complaining of weakness. Two patients were male, ages 72 and 50. The last four were females, between the ages of 24 and 40, all complaining of abdominal pain. It is 3:00 p.m. and time to restock the rooms. How many bedpans will you need?

- You are the primary nurse for an elderly patient with congestive heart failure. The IV stick was exceptionally difficult, but you are able to start an 18-gauge catheter on the second attempt. You leave the room to check on another patient. A relative thinks that the IV has stopped dripping and opens the clamp. How much IV fluid will infuse before you return?

- You have been asked to cover a coworker's rooms during her break. One of her patients is an elderly, confused male with an enlarged prostate. A catheter has been inserted and his physician is coming to see him. Somehow he manages to get off the stretcher. The drainage bag is firmly hooked to the side rail. Knowing that the catheter is 16 in. long and the drainage tubing is 3 ft long, will he be able to reach the door before pulling out the catheter?

Do you teach nursing documentation? Are you tired of trying to explain why it is important that the documentation is clear and accurate? Try using examples of what poor documentation can look like. Ask students what they think would happen if the following type of documentation were to be presented in court:

- The patient presented with left chest pain. Patient has chest pain if she lies on her left side for over a year.

- Healthy appearing decrepit 69-year-old male, mentally alert but forgetful admitted to room 304.

- The patient states she is numb from her toes down.

- When she fainted, her eyes rolled around the room.

When talking about the importance of patient teaching, one of the messages the instructor hopes the student hears is that it is important to be sure the patient understands the instructions or procedure. This understanding can be accomplished by asking the patient to either demonstrate the procedure or tell you what he or she has heard. To demonstrate this point, share a humorous situation. Here is an example:

A physician seeing a patient in the office found the patient's wound dressing to be extremely loose. When asked why the dressing was so loose, the patient explained, "Well, the nurse told me not to get the bandage wet, so whenever I take a shower, I take it off."

Flournoy, Turner, and Combs (2001) suggest using an interactive bulletin board to increase staff education in a critical care unit. The authors used humor to teach clinical concepts and found that certain components are necessary. First, there must be "a hook." Without something to draw people to the bulletin board, no matter how important the information, it will not be read. Then set up a pathway to follow, starting with the objectives, and create a smooth path with arrows leading to the information. The hook should be the "story line," which introduces the objective for the "lesson." Use a humorous story line by being creative. Perhaps a funny incident relates to the clinical topic. To be sure the story line will be effective, ask the following questions:

- Can this be misinterpreted by the participants?

- Will this offend participants?

- Will it decrease the author's credibility?

- Will it distract from the key points?

The second component is characters. Using cartoon characters is a suggestion. These can be hand drawn, computer clip art, or newspaper clippings. Use three principal characters: "One presents the information, one questions it, and one resists change" (p. 32cc8). The idea of resisting change is an interesting one, because experience shows that nurses may be reluctant to change viewpoints or ways of doing things. Resources for humorous healthcare cartoons include Nurstoon.com and JournalOfNursingJocularity.com.

The third component is the addition of diagrams, pathophysiology pictures, or statistical information. Learning requires a number of senses. Varying how the material is presented strengthens the delivery.

The fourth component is the post-test. Post-test questions relate to the clinical topic objectives. Berk (2002) suggests using a little humor in the test questions. Take the following example:

Ibuprofen is the generic drug name for which popular brand name medication?

1. Advil®
2. Black & Decker®
3. Charmin®
4. Docker®
5. Exxon®

Here is an example of how Flournoy, Turner, and Combs (2001) presented information on three different methods for obtaining a central venous pressure (CVP) measurement. The background color for the presentation was red because red is a powerful color and attracts attention. Numbered squares were used to indicate the flow of the story line. They used colored, computer-generated cartoon characters that included a reporter, office staff, and discharged patients who were visiting. Interaction between the characters was displayed through the use of speech bubbles. They designed a story in which the hospital office receives an announcement about three methods to obtain CVP. This announcement puts the office into a state of turmoil. A reporter from the *HitNurse Gazette* covers the story about this change. Through the use of diagrams, another character, named Calm Larry, explains how to implement the change. The story continues with some discussion by the cartoon characters about the need to change the way things are, and Smarty-Pants Mike explains the three methods that can be used. Brief questions are asked by the characters and Smarty-Pants Mike answers them. Then the reporter directs the participants to the post-test envelope. This particular training resulted in an average score of 90%.

Music and humor can assist the student in remembering information. There is a group called Too Live Nurse that includes performers whose job is to entertain as well as educate. One of their music productions is "Rockin' to the Algorithms" which is a music track that nurses have found helpful in preparing to pass their Advanced Cardiac Life Support (ACLS) examinations (Buxman, 2008). One nurse told Buxman (2008) that while she was taking the ACLS exam "I sang my way through it! It was funny, but I could remember the information because it was entertaining and I passed with flying colors!"

THE NEGATIVE SIDE OF HUMOR IN EDUCATION

A discussion of the use of humor for teaching purposes would not be complete without discussing the problems that can occur when humor is used inappropriately. Some people feel that humor has no place in education and may become offended if humor is used in the classroom or in patient education. When using humor, be sensitive to the responses of the student or students. Any humor that puts someone down should not be used. In reality, that is not humor but an insult. As Boerman-Cornell (2000) said, "Humor that hurts the audience is counterproductive" (¶20). Hurtful humor stifles creativity and learner participation and creates an atmosphere of fear.

CASE STUDY

Martha, the social worker from hospice, was asked to share her knowledge about therapeutic humor to the caregivers of the hospice patients. She felt honored to do this and took the task very seriously because she felt it was important for others to understand how important laughter and humor were for the caregivers and their loved ones who were dying.

Questions

1. What visual aids can she use to humorously augment the information shared?

2. What things would she need to be cautious of when using humor in her lecture?

3. How would she know if her humor was effective?

Discussion

As Martha is preparing for this presentation, it would be helpful for her to be alert for cartoons or funny stories that she can use to add to the talk. Doing a PowerPoint with some cute graphics would be an attention getter. Being careful to use color and wording carefully so that the slides are not too busy is also important. Adding funny comments, or even talking with an accent, if appropriate, can catch a learner's attention. Martha needs to be sure the comments are not sarcastic or offensive. There are some activities she could use to get the audience involved, if there is time to do that. Things can be done to make people aware of the changes that occur when you go from frowning to smiling. For physiological changes, she can have someone in the audience volunteer to come up on stage and have them demonstrate what it looks like when someone laughs, and as she talks, she can start laughing also. Soon most, if not all, the audience will be laughing and experiencing the feelings themselves. Then she can talk about what they felt. It is important for her to stay alert to the body language of the participants. If she notices someone is offended, she might need to address that. Her ability to "read" the audience will give her some idea of the effectiveness of the presentation. She can also ask for questions and gauge the change of understanding by the questions asked. A formal evaluation asking for a rating of the presentation, material, and presenter might also be helpful in evaluating the effectiveness of the program.

SUMMARY

Learning is an ongoing process. Many theories address how people learn; however, no one theory covers all the aspects of learning. Individuals learn based on their genetic background, psychological and physical well-being, and the opportunities that they encounter. Developmental issues affect the learning process. Most people become increasingly self-directed as they age. Nurses can assist the learner by being aware of the learner's style, developmental level, innate ability, and recent research in the field of knowledge acquisition.

There is strong evidence that humor has a place in education, whether it be patient education or nursing education. Raseshide (1993, cited in Flowers, 2001) suggests seven guidelines for using humor in the classroom. These guidelines serve as a good summary for humor in education, no matter what the environment.

- Be aware of and receptive to the many uses of humor.

- Never use humor to ridicule or embarrass the learner.

- Humor should serve a specific purpose, even if it is used spontaneously.

- Humor should be appropriate to the learner's ability level.

- Spontaneous and planned humor should be used in teaching.

- People should laugh at themselves occasionally to demonstrate that they are real people.

- Sarcasm should only be used if it is playful, and even then it should be used very carefully. It should be noted that some students find sarcasm inappropriate and hurtful.

EXAM QUESTIONS

CHAPTER 11
Questions 80-86

Note: Choose the one option that BEST answers each question.

80. A nurse-manager is planning an in-service session to teach the staff how to use a new IV pump. She designs the program using cartoons and dresses up the IV pole as a clown. This type of approach will probably

    a. cause staff ridicule.

    b. make the administration uncomfortable.

    c. lose the interest of the learner.

    d. increase the interest and attention of the learner.

81. A healthcare provider plans on teaching her newly diagnosed cardiac patient about potential lifestyle changes necessary to improve his cardiovascular health. She decides to add humor into the teaching process. Adding humor is a way to

    a. decrease tension so that learning is more likely to take place.

    b. increase tension, thereby increasing creativity.

    c. emphasize the importance of lifestyle changes that are necessary.

    d. help patients laugh at themselves.

82. Using cartoons in a preoperative teaching booklet

    a. helps increase comprehension.

    b. always guarantees compliance.

    c. makes the booklet more difficult to read.

    d. insults adults and should be avoided.

83. Negative reinforcement of behaviors, such as repeatedly saying "no" or "bad," is an example of

    a. rationalism.

    b. social learning.

    c. inactive learning.

    d. operant conditioning.

84. A nurse is preparing to teach a 76-year-old woman how to administer her own insulin. The most important principle to keep in mind during the instruction for this patient is that

    a. older adults cannot learn new information.

    b. humor for an older adult is distracting and should never be used.

    c. using humor that taps into former knowledge is helpful.

    d. learning methods do not need to be adjusted for age.

85. In order to increase learning through use of humor, which of the following strategies should be considered?

    a. Use funny but relevant visual aids.

    b. Make jokes about other people.

    c. Always include funny stories.

    d. Develop the ability to tell jokes well.

86. A negative type of humor in teaching that should be avoided is

    a. laughing at yourself occasionally.

    b. to ridicule or embarrass the learner.

    c. the use of empathetic humor.

    d. spontaneous humor with a purpose.

CHAPTER 12

DESIGNING HUMOR PROGRAMS IN WORK SETTINGS

CHAPTER OBJECTIVE

After completing this chapter, the reader will be able to describe different types of formal humor programs and the concerns and considerations related to implementing such a program.

LEARNING OUTCOMES

After studying the chapter, the reader will be able to

1. explain different types of humor projects.
2. design a humor project.
3. create a humor program in his or her facility.
4. discuss the role of caring clowns.
5. explain how someone might become involved in care clowning.

INTRODUCTION

Not only is it important to understand the benefits of humor, it is also important to find ways to add humor to everyday experiences. A number of formal methods can be used to accomplish this, such as the use of humor rooms, humor carts, or humor baskets. Caring clowns is another means of intervention. This chapter explores formal methods of introducing humor into your life and the lives of patients and coworkers.

HUMOR PROJECTS

Commonly used types of humor projects include humor rooms, humor carts, humor baskets, and caring clowns.

Humor Rooms

Humor rooms are rooms where patients, family, friends, and staff can get together to laugh, play, and relax. These rooms are commonly decorated with comfortable furniture, pleasing artwork, and plants. One of the first humor rooms created was "The Lively Room" at DeKalb Hospital in Decatur, Georgia (Buxman, 1991; Gibson, 1995; Wooten, 1996). It was started by Sandra Yates, RN, and W.W. Lively, a hospital board member.

Humor rooms usually contain reading areas, video equipment, and shelves filled with humorous books, videos, audiocassettes, and other materials. If the room is large enough, it can be used as a place for informal gatherings, group sessions, and even birthday parties or weddings.

The negative side of a humor room is that it is stationary. Patients from other areas of a hospital have limited access to it. In addition, it is difficult for patients who are seriously ill or bedridden to access the materials in the room. Humor rooms work well in long-term care facilities, rehabilitation units, psychiatric units, and outpatient clinics (Wooten, 1996).

Humor Carts

Humor carts can be filled with the same materials and supplies as humor rooms. However, carts can be wheeled into a patient's room to brighten the somber, scary, stress-filled days that go along with hospital admissions. In 1989, Leslie Gibson, RN, created one of the first humor carts at Morton Plant Hospital in Clearwater, Florida. Some of the items she suggests included in a humor cart are books, comics, and magazines, a surprise box with such items as funny glasses, animal noses, masks, puppets, gags, and card games, a collection of cartoons; and portable tape recorders and humorous cassettes (Gibson, 1995). If the budget allows, a DVD player in a locking portable cabinet with DVDs can add hours of enjoyment for patients. Some televisions come in combination with DVD players.

Wooten (1995) mentions that carts can be different shapes and sizes. Some places use carts that look like old library carts. Others use big red toolboxes on wheels that are full of drawers and cabinets that can be locked. If a big red toolbox on wheels is used, Wooten (1995) suggests decorating it so that it does not look like a crash cart.

Patti Bihn, RN, received a grant from the *Journal of Nursing Jocularity* to create a humor cart for the intensive care unit (ICU) at St. Joseph Mercy Hospital in Ann Arbor, Michigan. In sharing her struggle to start a humor cart, Bihn (1995) offers ideas that can help others find carts and gather equipment. Bihn searched for something inexpensive to use as a cart. She tried to get one donated but could not. She finally got a cart with six baskets in a rolling metal frame. After she obtained the cart, the next step was to fill it. Bihn (1995) shares what she included in her cart (Table 12-1).

Terry Bennett, an oncology nurse, helped start a humor cart at the Fox Chase Cancer Center in Philadelphia (Wooten, 1995). She found the nursing administration supportive of the effort, but the hospital administration was not as enthusiastic. To

TABLE 12-1: EXAMPLES OF CONTENTS INCLUDED IN A HUMOR CART

- Modeling compound
- Rolls of smiley heart stickers
- Crossword puzzle books
- Videos and audiocassettes
- Fake poop in a specimen container (some of the props are to share with staff as well as with patients)
- Playing cards
- Slide puzzles
- Slinky
- Pinwheel head boppers (these are "pinwheels attached to a headband and make an interesting sight when transferring a patient out of the unit") [p. 33]
- Plastic duckies
- Silly apparel, such as witch hats, jester clothing, and goofy hats
- Gold cardboard crowns and tinsel (which can be used for a patient's birthday or some other special event)
- Rubber chicken (no cart is complete without such an item)
- Giant clown scissors and glasses
- Bubbles
- Back scratchers

(Bihn, 1995)

convince them of the usefulness of the project, articles and news clippings about the benefits of humor and health were presented. With permission granted, she gathered her materials from many of the local retailers in the community. She wrote letters requesting donations and received many positive responses.

In an interview with Wooten (1995), Bennett shared that the most popular item among cancer patients was a video by Joe Kogel called *Life and Depth*. Kogel is a cancer survivor who gives a funny presentation about using humor to maintain a positive attitude and keep up hopes. Bennett also found that some contemporary videos were enjoyed. *Wayne's World* was a preferred video among adolescents, and seniors preferred such actors as Charlie Chaplin, Buster Keaton, and Lucille Ball. She also noted that having some audiotapes and videotapes of peaceful environments, such as meadowlands or seashores, were appreciated.

Laugh Mobile

Research has spurred the use of humor programs in hospital settings. One such program is the "Laugh Mobile," developed by Ruth Hamilton, the founder of the Carolina Health and Humor Association (Carolina Ha Ha). The "Laugh Mobile" is part of the Duke University Medical Center Humor Project, a joint venture between Carolina Ha Ha and Duke Oncology Recreational Therapy, that was started in 1987 (Hamilton, 2003). The "Laugh Mobile" is a humor cart that takes materials to inpatient and outpatient cancer patients. Since its initial development, a new "Laugh Mobile" has been developed and is being marketed to medical facilities nationwide.

Humor Baskets

Humor baskets have smaller numbers of items than humor carts and humor rooms. They are commonly used by family caregivers to bring humor into the lives of loved ones who are at home. Wooten (1996) writes about one nurse, Cathy Johnson of Dartmouth-Hitchcock Medical Center in Lyme, New Hampshire, who felt a need to improve the mood of patients enduring lengthy hospitalizations and prolonged bed rest. Not having much financial backing, she found a large wicker basket that she filled with assorted toys and gadgets.

A fun addition to a humor basket is medicine bottles filled with humorous comments. Wooten (1996) suggests that it is a good idea to place jokes for different age-groups and genders into different jars and label them. This way, jokes that would more likely be of interest for a certain group can be easily found. Finding one-liners to place in the bot-

tles can be fun and offers a lighthearted touch to the seriousness of illness. Some suggestions for one-liners are:

- I intend to live forever – so far, so good.
- When everything is coming your way, you're in the wrong lane.
- When I'm in my right mind, my left mind gets pretty crowded.
- Energizer Bunny arrested; charged with battery.
- Shin: a device for finding furniture in the dark.
- Laughing stock: cattle with a sense of humor.
- One of the great blessings about living in a democracy is that we have complete control over how we pay our taxes…cash, check, credit card or money order.

Caring Clowns

No one expects a clown to be profound. No one expects a clown to be anything but funny. Look again! The clown will catch you off guard and speak directly to your heart – make you laugh at yourself and weep with the world.

– Shobi Dobi, CLL

Caring clowns are clowns who work in various areas of health care, such as hospitals, long-term care facilities, and home care. They are usually people who are specially trained to be sensitive to the needs of sick people. Patty Wooten is a well-known clown who is also an RN. She states that caring clowns should be "sensitive, be able to read nonverbal body language, and possess good listening skills" (Wooten, 1992, p. 46).

In an article on clowning Dr. Patch Adams (2002) states, "Clowning needs to be context, not a therapy…Of course it is therapeutic" (p. 9). Clowning is Adams' way of bringing love and joy to patients.

Jenny Thompson-Richards, MSW (2006) is a caring clown who does her healing work at a hospice in Australia with two other caring clowns. She shares her view of what caring clowns do.

We articulate some of the why is and how is of caring clowning. Clown Doctors aim to affirm people as people with richly storied lives, to give permission for both laughter and tears, and to bring consolation to the spirit. The art of clowning means that we seek to elevate people, to sensitively tailor music, touch, and color to the interests of those we encounter, to invite a sense of wonder and spontaneity and to work to transform situations through the imagination.

People commonly think of clowns being used in pediatrics, and indeed they are, but they can be a beneficial diversion for people of all ages. At one of the annual American Association for Therapeutic Humor (AATH) conferences, a person who acts as a mime in nursing homes had a running video of her experience working in a long-term care facility. One clip showed her working with a woman with dementia. The woman looked confused and disoriented at first. The mime sat down next to her and slowly drew her out. Toward the end of the clip, she was kidding along with the mime and smiling.

Selena Clare McMahan (2008) shares her experiences in South Africa with an organization called Clowns Without Borders. Although much of her time as a caring clown was spent working with children, some of her most poignant experiences were working with the elderly. At one town, while doing work with orphanages and children's hospitals, they were housed in an "old-age home." They volunteered to perform for their "housemates." In comparison to the loud, joyous laughter of children, they found the laughter of adults to be slow in coming and less explosive, but "they had a kind of a depth that the children's laughter never reached" (p. 21). They brought members of the audience up on stage and they tended to be the funniest volunteers. The residents were very verbal about their appreciation for the clowns and the joy they brought, and the memories they triggered.

McMahan found that clowning with the elderly, meeting them where they were physically and emotionally and helping them find playfulness at a time when life does not hold joy, brings a satisfaction and sense of wonder she found very moving.

In 2001, a mortuary in the Phoenix area employed Eloise Cole as a bereavement specialist. What makes her unique is that she is a clown who uses her clown character, Rainbow, to help clients deal with fears, questions, guilt, and other emotions that are part of the grieving process. Cole (2001) shared her development of Rainbow with the audience at the 2001 AATH conference.

Rainbow was developed when Cole realized that she was heard in a different way when she used humor to talk about serious topics. She found that people tended to let down their defenses and hear what she was saying when humor was part of the process. Through her exploration of the use of humor, she became interested in the art of clowning. Rainbow offers a way for people to get in touch with their grief experience on an emotional level. Cole (2001) explains the process of Rainbow's development and work this way:

> I chose the name of Rainbow for the symbolism. I put together a 12-minute presentation that encapsulates some of the major dynamics of the mourning experience. Rainbow appears as a happy clown and then tells her audience a story from a time in her life when she was really down because someone she loved had died.

> Using a variety of props, Rainbow talks about the pain of someone dying, the efforts to be strong and keep busy, and feeling crazy. She uses props such as a feather duster for keeping busy, a world globe symbolizes carrying the weight of the world on her shoulders, and a crab puppet symbolizes feeling crabby and out of sorts. Rainbow moves through some of the elements of mourning and then realizes that

she needs help. Again props are used to point out the need for rest and nutrition and the avoidance of alcohol and drugs. Rainbow then asks for help and for people to listen to her and her pain. She discovers that she can learn to change, grow, and find new rainbows.

One of the best-known caring clown projects is the Big Apple Circus Clown Care Unit which started in New York City (Wooten, 1996). The project is made up of professional clowns who visit pediatric patients. The program started in 1986 in New York after the death of the cofounder's brother. It has expanded to include at least 17 hospitals across the country (Yale-New Haven Children's Hospital, 2002). In 1996, the Hinda and Richard Rosenthal Center for Complementary and Alternative Medicine at Columbia University in New York presented a $150,000 grant for the study of the impact of clown therapy on children's well-being. The purpose of the grant was to investigate the effect clown visits have on decreasing physiological and psychological distress in children and adolescents during clinical procedures.

Three different reports are posted on the Rosenthal Center Web site concerning the results of the Clown Care Unit studies. Two of the studies discussed were pilot studies (Gorfinkle, Slater, Bagiella, Tager, & Labinsky, 1998, Balick & Lee, 2003). One study looked at the effect of clowns on children undergoing venipunctures, infusaport access, intramuscular injection, or lumbar puncture. The children were ages 3 to 18 and were randomly assigned to clown visits at either visit 1 or visit 2. The results of this study showed no significant difference in observed child distress with the clown present. The doctors and nurses, however, found the procedures easier to perform when the clowns were present.

In the second study, 28 heart transplant recipients ages 6 to 20 were observed during two consecutive biopsies in a cardiac catheterization laboratory. During their second visit, participants were assigned to a clown or no-clown situation. Children who were exposed to the clowns showed a marginally significant decrease in observed child distress and a significant decrease in child self-reported distress. There was also a significant decrease in parent-rated child distress. However, these results failed to reach significance when baseline differences were covaried. In addition, doctors found the procedure more difficult to perform with the clowns present (Gorfinkle et al., 1998; Balick & Lee, 2003).

The results of the third study indicate a significant decrease in observed child distress, child-reported distress, and parent-rated child distress when clowns were present during cardiac catheterization. Positive changes were seen in hospital caregivers' behavior and mood when the clowns were around. The clowns were introduced to three new hospitals for this study, and all of them remained at the conclusion of the study (Gorfinkle et al., 1998; Balick & Lee, 2003).

"I've decided to cure illness with a little humor!"

Note. From DansCartoons.com. Used with permission.

Developing a Caring Clown

Wooten (1996) found her inner clown in 1973 and started developing her clown characters soon after. Learning to be a clown is an educational process, and there are schools devoted to that purpose. Wooten started her clown training with a Ringling Brothers Clown College graduate who was teaching a "clownology" course through San Diego State University. She started out with Scruffy the Clown and later developed Nancy Nurse. Nancy Nurse is a wild, redheaded clown who comes decked out with a combat belt filled with weapons, such as a bedpan, a urinal, an enema bucket, and over-sized syringes. She wears a stethoscope made from a garden hose with a toilet plunger, which she says "is great to use on those big-hearted patients…it can also be used to relieve constipation" (Wooten, 1996, p. 144). She is bold and outspoken and controls doctors and nurses. Her character is funny and nurses love her outrageous behavior and solutions to common problems. When asked to visit patients, however, Wooten learned that Nurse Nancy could be a little too bold and too boisterous for patients and their families. So guideline number one, make sure the character fits the purpose of the job.

In 1994, Nurse Kindheart, a sweet, white-haired nurse with a proper British accent was born. Nurse Kindheart demonstrates patience and kindness as she visits those in need of ministering. Being aware of the needs and reactions of patients and their families caused Wooten to develop this antithesis to Nancy Nurse. The contrast of the two clowns is distinct, with Nurse Nancy bringing tears of laughter, and Nurse Kindheart causing a feeling of comfortable amusement. The development of the right clown, like the development of a person as they travel through life, depends on the circumstances, the personality of the performer, and the sensitivity of the person from whom the clown develops.

Wooten (1996) suggests guidelines for clown visitations in Table 12-2.

So You Want to Be a Clown

Are you already a clown or would you like to take lessons to become more knowledgeable about clowning? If this area of caring interests you, attend training. There are a number of clown schools throughout the United States. *The Hospital Clown Newsletter* at http://www.hospitalclown.com offers suggestions, shares ideas, and gives general support. Letting out the clown in you allows you to put more joy into your life and into the lives of others. Patty Wooten, in her book *Compassionate Laughter: Jest for Your Health,* has two chapters on clowning. One chapter offers ideas for different ways to present yourself.

TABLE 12-2: GUIDELINES FOR CLOWN VISITATIONS

- Visits should be pre-approved and scheduled.
- Visits should occur between 9 a.m. and 8 p.m.
- Clowns should check in at the nursing station and obtain feedback about and suggestions for patient visits.
- Clowns should request the staff to accompany them to the patient's room on the first visit.
- Prior to entering the room, clowns should request permission from the patient to visit.
- Clowns should not move patients or manipulate hospital equipment. The staff should be called if necessary.
- Gifts should be approved by the staff before being given to patients.
- Visits should be limited to 10 minutes, unless staff permits longer visits.
- Clowns should stop at the nursing station after visits are completed to obtain any other requests or notify the staff that they are leaving.

(Wooten, 1996)

The story in Table 12-3, from *The Hospital Clown Newsletter* at http://www.hospitalclown.com, portrays the essence of what a hospital clown does. The clown stays in character, reaches out with his or her heart, brings joy and comfort to those around him or her, and then finds a way to let go of the sorrows and burdens of others.

Dr. Patch Adams (2002) believes all members of a hospital staff should think about being clowns. He feels that thinking about clowning (or humor, love, and joy) as therapy and the clown as a specialist who does the clowning might lead others to think they do not have to help bring love, humor, or joy to the patient. He states, "I want to put in an encouragement for each person, professional clown or not, to imagine that what they do each day can be a potent part of creating a context of love and fun" (Adams, 2002, p. 17). He contends that, if each of us brought joy and comfort to those around us, our jobs would be more rewarding and those around us would experience less suffering.

Bringing Clowns into a Facility

With all of the literature available on the importance of humor and with the development of caring clown programs, one would think that healthcare facility administrations would be thrilled to have someone offer to start such a program. This is often not the case. Shobhana Schwebke (n.d.), who goes by the clown name Shobie Dobie and is the editor of *The Hospital Clown Newsletter,* feels that part of the problem is an administration's need to put clowns in hospital categories. She states, "Hospital care is a scientific-based discipline; the clown is a heart-based discipline" (p. 3). Approaching an administration can be a challenge. Wooten (1996) offers the following suggestions:

- The first visit to a hospital or nursing home should be done wearing street clothes.

- Meet with appropriate staff (for example, the child development specialist or nursing supervisor).

- Obtain permission and establish guidelines. (Be sure to bring suggestions with you because many facilities do not have guidelines for entertainers who visit patients.)

- Present a professional manner.

- Convince the administration of your intent to work with the system to develop a program that will benefit the facility and the patients.

THE PLANNING STAGES

Humor rooms, humor carts, comedy via closed-circuit television, and hospital clowns are all examples of how to bring therapeutic humor into a facility. Whatever type of program a facility wants to implement, it takes time and money to put it all together. Convincing the administration of the importance of adding humor to the hospital environment may also take time and effort. After all, hospitals are about serious business. Using research to support your argument can help convince the administration that humor can be an inexpensive tool to increase patient health and satisfaction with the care they receive.

When planning a project, keep in mind the audience for the humor. If the audience is very young children or older adults, DVDs and cassette tapes may need to be shorter to accommodate shorter attention spans. Cultural issues are also an important consideration. Are most of the patients in the facility Mexican, Cuban, or African American? Can you get material that would be of interest to that cultural group? These are questions to consider. Throughout the process, thought and careful planning are essential.

Getting Started

It is a good idea to form a committee of people who are interested in providing some type of humor program in your facility. It is suggested to include someone from pastoral care, a volunteer from the volunteer program, someone from the

TABLE 12-3: I LOVE YOU WOLLIE

(as told to Shobi by Jackie Garner)

I was packing to go to a convention when I got a call from a hospital I'd never been to. I don't know how they found out about Lolli. They said "We have a little boy in ICU. Could you come as fast as you can?" I had already packed my costume, but when I heard ICU, I had Lolli clowned up and at that hospital in 30 minutes. I had never and never since put on my makeup that fast. I could never makeup again that fast or that well except that it was something that I was called to do.

I get up to Pediatric ICU and as soon as the elevator doors open you can hear crying and moaning cause these kids don't like being there and they're hurting. Now ICU is normally glassed rooms, because they have to be able to see everything. You can see all the children in their beds. You haven't been called to see them, but all those children are watching you. So I go into a little boy's room – his name was Vincent. He is four and a half years old. And again you could hear moaning. I come around the corner and in character voice say "Hello." The doctor says, "You must be Lolli!" "Yes, and who is this handsome boy?" The doctor introduces "This is Vincent." Lolli continues "Are you married? Are you engaged to anyone?" He doesn't say anything, he is just looking at me, but his eyes are smiling. He's not scared of me after all he's four and one-half.

The doctor says, "Lolli, do you mind if we bring in a rocking chair? Would you like to sit in a rocking chair and hold Vincent?" Lolli answered "Sure would." So, they brought in this beautiful white rocking chair. And again I can be seen by all the other children all around me from their beds. They lay a pad across my lap and they lay Vincent in my arms, and he is so close. His eyes immediately go to my jeweled heart nose. He's checking out my hair, my face and all the bright colors. And Mama is looking right over my left shoulder and Daddy's looking right over my right shoulder, so we are all close. "Lolli loves you, Vincent."

I can tell he wants to touch my nose. So I take his finger and push my nose and laugh. "This is little Lolli's laugh button. Tee hee, Little Lolli loves you, Vincent." Mama's over the left shoulder saying "I love you, baby" and Daddy says "It's O.K. son, Daddy's here."

About 30 minutes goes by – just quiet time of giggles and nose pushing. In that time I knew this child like my own. We made a connection that no one could ever separate. Yet, he had not said one word to me. All of a sudden, Vincent pushes my nose again and he giggles all the way to his toes. Just giggles. Not one tear. There was no pain. This is what happens, something magical happens when a clown is there with a child in a one-on-one.

He just had the sweetest smile in his eyes and face. And each time I would say "Little Lolli loves you, Vincent," and Mama and Daddy would say "I'm here, I love you." This time I pushed my nose and giggled and said, "I love you." He took a breath and spoke, "I love you, Wollie." I wanted to change my name to Wollie, right there. Then he said "I love you, Mommy. I love you, Daddy." And with this, his eyes went up to my eyes and my nose. "You want to push my nose again." So I took his little finger and pushed my nose. As I said "Little Lolli loves you, Vincent," he takes in the deepest breath, his smile broadens and his eyes are glistening. Then he breathes out his last breath. He dies in Lolli's arms.

The doctor comes over and takes Vincent from my arms and the mother and father go with him and I'm thinking, I've got to get out of here. I've got to run. But I look up at all those kids around me. They don't know what just happened. They are watching my every move. I am the clown. I am not Jackie Garner dressed as Lollibelle - I am Lolli to them. I am the only clown they may ever see. So I wave "Hello" in Lolli's character voice, but I'm thinking I've got to get out of here. I go out the door and there is a child right there. "Hello, Lolli loves you." I'm thinking, if I can just get to the elevator, I can let this out. I'm half way down the hall and I can see the elevator button. "Hello, Hi" waving to the other children. Inside me, the mother I am, is screaming, but these kids don't see this. It does not show on my face, because I am Little Lolli the clown.

Jackie Garner cannot do this. God has a part in this, something greater has control of this for you when you do this with all your heart and you want to help the kids. He's going to help you do it. That's the only way you are going to get through it. I'm not a great person. I'm not superwoman. I just have to let go and let Him help me handle it.

So, I'm almost to the elevator, and here come Vincent's Dad. "Clown, wait!" Tears are running down his face and he is reaching into his pocket. "What do I owe you?" I answer softly "Nothing, what do I owe you?" And I leaned over and whispered into his ear. "There are children watching and I have to stay in clown character." And as I go to the elevator I wave. "I love you, Daddy. Bye! Bye!" I push the button and I see the down light flashing, but here comes the mother crying. "Lolli, please I need to see you." I answer in character "Okay, Mom." And I think that was the longest walk I ever made in my life – back down the hall toward the mother. When I get there, Mom just falls into my arms – and she is sobbing into my costume – and I can feel her tears go past my hair and down my neck. "Lolli, he never got to go to Disney World, my baby never even got to see the circus and all of that. Oh, did you notice the way he went, there was no pain. He was smiling, he was giggling." And Lolli whispered in her ear, "I know, Mom. He's going to be fine. You're going to see him someday and you're going to take up just where you left off. But other children are watching Lolli. I love you and from one mommy to another I do understand. Thank you for letting me be a part of this." She looked up, "We will never forget you, Lolli." Daddy comes out and they walk back down the hall. And there I am trying to get back to the elevator, again, in character waving to the children "Hello, Hi, Little Lolli loves you." The children for all they knew, the child fell asleep in my arms.

The elevator door opens and sure enough there was a mom inside with two kids. "Hello!" I'm thinking, soon I'll be outside and I can let go. And the lobby was full of kids, and the parking lot looked like Disney World. "Hello! How ya doing?" I get on the freeway and everyone is driving by waving at the clown – "Oh look there is a clown. Hello, Clown." I'm thinking, God find me a dirt road please! And I found one right after I asked for it. I drove down that road and there wasn't a soul on the road and I was able to let go and cry. These to me are the true tears of a clown. When you are touched by something and you realize that you are being used to touch and offer healing. Be it death or whatever, you never know what you are going to be asked to do.

Note. From The Hospital Clown Newsletter, *Retrieved June 3, 2010, from http://www.hospitalclown.com/InfoPages/storiesTable.htm. Reprinted with permission.*

nursing department, someone from physical therapy or occupational therapy, a social service person, and someone from administration (Buxman, 1991, Gibson, 1995). When one person bears all the responsibility, if that person leaves or becomes overwhelmed, the project may cease. Spreading responsibility decreases the potential for failure.

Once the committee has been organized, it is time to think about what the committee would like to see developed with the resources that might be available. Having knowledge of what other facilities have done to bring humor to their patients or residents (in the case of long-term care facilities) can help identify possibilities. Gibson (1995) cautions that the committee should go slow and not try to serve everybody in the beginning. She recommends starting on one unit and getting the staff and patients motivated on that unit.

Cost Concerns

To help determine how much the project will cost, it is necessary to brainstorm. A good starting place would be to think about:

- where or what will be used, such as the waiting room, humor baskets, or humor carts.

- how to designate the area.

- what type of program the facility can afford.

- where financing might be available.

- how the facility will advertise the program.

- where materials might come from.

Think about what materials the program will have to pay for and what materials might be available from staff, patients, and the community. The most popular items for comedy carts, humor rooms, and baskets are humorous DVDs or audiotapes, cartoon albums, humorous books, gag items, and props such as Groucho glasses or clowns' noses.

Obtaining funding might require some creativity. Gibson (1995) recommends contacting the local Rotary, Kiwanis, and Women's Leagues to ask them to sponsor a program at your facility. Contact local merchants to see if they would be willing to donate equipment, videos, or books. Contact the volunteer committee of the hospital and see if volunteers would be willing to have a fundraiser to raise money for the project. One hospital in Pennsylvania put an advertisement in the local newspaper asking for humorous items (Gibson, 1995). They ended up receiving thousands of items.

Some hospitals have applied to the Humor Project, a program in Saratoga Springs, New York, founded and directed by Joel Goodman, for humor research grants to start programs. In 1996, Intergris Baptist Hospital Medical Center in Oklahoma City started a Medical Institute for Recovery Through Humor (MIRTH) program in its 20-bed skilled nursing facility (Foltz-Gray, 1998). Goodman went to the facility to do an hour-long training session. The Humor Project offered MIRTH a $3,000 grant to start the project, which serves as a research vehicle, a humor resource center, and a place of support for patients, family, and staff.

Advertising

In order for a project to work, people need to know about it. Having a name for the project is helpful. Communication about the project is important. Suggested means of advertising the project include calling the press, putting information about the project in the hospital newsletter, and having a party to celebrate the opening of the project (Gibson, 1995). Talk about the project in staff meetings, and make sure that the physicians know about it. Get creative. The more people who know about the project, the more likely it is to be successful.

Supplies

Storing supplies can be a challenge. Hospitals are always looking for new places to store things. In the beginning, a cart that can be locked might be the best idea, unless a room is available. The cart can be placed somewhere visible, decorated with bright colors, and labeled so people know what it is. This tactic serves as another form of advertising as well as a place to store the humor equipment.

The program must have a method to account for and monitor the supplies. Gibson (1995) learned that people did not always return items that were used, and supplies disappeared. Designing a sign-out sheet is a good precautionary measure. The sheet can include the name of the person who uses the material, the department or room number, the resource taken (such as game, magazine, or DVD), and a place to sign it back into the supply area.

Having an inventory of the supplies is important. Gibson (1995) suggests putting numbers on books, videos, and cassette tapes so that they can be cataloged. Doing so also helps keep a record of what you have. Cataloging also makes it easier for patients to know what is available. Utilize volunteers to help with this duty.

Supplies may be obtained through a number of sources. Bihn (1995) shares her experience of gathering supplies for a humor cart for the intensive care unit at St. Joseph Mercy Hospital in Ann Arbor, Michigan. Some of the supplies were ordered from various companies, but she was also able to obtain donations from a local video store and a novelty store. The video store donated three comedies, and the novelty store donated a rubber chicken, jumbo sunglasses, and jumbo scissors.

Training

Training the volunteers and staff who will work with the humor program and providing inservice programs on the humor project are important. The volunteers who will work with the program need to be oriented to hospital policies and to the lay out of the facility.

In addition, the people who are working with the program need to know their roles (Gibson, 1995). Guidelines regarding expectations need to be developed and included in the training sessions. As volunteers start to work, keep them busy so they do not get bored, especially in the beginning of the program (Gibson, 1995). Encourage them to sit with or play checkers with patients to promote involvement.

Volunteers need to know that not everyone will be interested or feel well enough to participate in humor activities. They also need to know that they should not touch patients or be loud, especially if they are acting as clowns. Discourage volunteers from asking, "How are you today?" because "we want to divert [patients] from the 'poor me' angle" (Gibson, 1995, p. 122). Instead, encourage them to ask, "What can I offer you today?" Those involved in the humor project must understand that humor should not be forced on anybody.

HUMORING THE STAFF

The previously mentioned interventions discuss ways to bring humor to patients, but what about the staff? Hospital staff is under a lot of stress on a daily basis. Nursing staff members are often overworked and work in difficult situations. The present nursing shortage adds to the normal stress of caring for people who are seriously ill or may be dying, fearful, or in pain. Adding humor to a staff's daily working environment can help increase morale, improve relations between different departments, and help decrease the stress level.

Some hospitals have used humor during the celebration of nurses' week. A small hospital in southwestern Arizona contacted three nurses who called themselves the Ha Ha Sisterhood to come in and do something on humor and health for the nursing staff. These three nurses started out presenting the program for the local community college. One nurse was an emergency room supervisor, and the other two nurses were educators at the local community college. They came together periodically to educate and share the joy of humor. The program offered nurses a chance to laugh, let their hair down, and let go of the stresses of the day. For example, before one program started, a member of the dietary staff borrowed one of the wigs and had a fun time laughing and sharing with her coworkers.

Nurses have also been known to take items off of their facility's humor cart to use with fellow staff members to lighten the daily load. Another way to introduce humor into the work environment is to place a bulletin board at the nurses' station or in the area where staff congregate with space for sharing cartoons, puns, and jokes. One effective way for healthcare providers to find stress release is to generate and share in humorous situations. Doing so does not make the care provider unprofessional, as some may think; rather, it increases creativity and boosts morale.

CASE STUDY

*F*our members of the healthcare team were sitting around talking about the need to increase humor on the bone marrow transplant floor. Patients receiving bone marrow transplant may range from toddlers to aged adults. Other patients are admitted to this floor, but all rooms can be converted for patients undergoing bone marrow transplants. The four members were a staff nurse, the social worker, a child-life worker, and the infection control nurse. Many ideas were brought up and some were discarded, others were put in the "maybe this will work" basket, and others were in the "yes, that is a great idea" basket.

Questions

1. Whose buy-in do they need to make this work?

2. What are the possible approaches to gather financial and other support for this project?

3. What kinds of concerns will they have in this particular unit?

Discussion

The members of the group decide that they need to first approach the unit coordinator to assure her support in the process of implementing a program. If the staff receives support and encouragement from medical staff, the unit coordinator/charge nurse, and other members of the healthcare team, they can then approach administrators and board members. To gather support they need to review and present research articles that support their hypothesis that adding humor materials and making them available to patients will improve patient outcomes. They also need to think about where they might get financial support, and contact a few key people to ascertain if they might be able to help fund the program. Some potential areas of support are community organizations such as Rotary or Kiwanis. The hospital volunteer organization often helps raise money for specific areas or equipment in the hospital; possible grants may be available through organizations that support cancer patients. Sometimes local retailers are willing to help with materials, so contacting places such as Sears, Wal-Mart, Kmart, or even Spencers might yield materials or financial help. The committee will also need to think about the type of equipment and materials they might use. Because the patients on this unit are highly susceptible to infection, ways of sanitizing or at least cleaning the materials used is important. If they decide on using caring clowns, they will need to be sure education is offered that emphasizes cleanliness and hand washing. Another thing this group might need is enthusiasm, "stick-to-itism," and lots of humor.

SUMMARY

There are a number of ways to provide humor intervention in medical facilities. Humor rooms, humor carts, and humor baskets are three common examples. Caring clowns are specially trained people who can bring laughter and play to those who are ill. Whatever humor intervention is used, it takes time and energy to develop a program, but patients benefit from the experience in immeasurable ways.

The lessons from this chapter are:

- There are different types of humor projects:
    - Humor rooms
    - Humor Carts
    - Humor Baskets
    - Caring Clowns
- Humor projects do not just happen; they take planning and work.
- Planning stages of humor projects include:
    - getting people, especially administration, to support the idea;
    - brain storming what will work in the facility;
    - obtaining funding sources;
    - finding the materials or persons needed;
    - educating and training staff.
- Don't forget the staff – the staff needs humor too.
    - Create bulletin boards for cartoons and jokes.
    - Create theme days such as crazy hat day or a humor day.

EXAM QUESTIONS

CHAPTER 12
Questions 87-93

Note: Choose the one option that BEST answers each question.

87. The difference between a humor cart and a humor room is

    a. humor carts have DVDs in them and humor rooms do not.

    b. humor rooms are easier to supply than humor carts.

    c. humor rooms have props, such as clown noses, and humor carts do not.

    d. humor carts are mobile and provide greater patient access.

88. According to oncology nurse Terry Bennett, a good DVD to have in a humor cart is

    a. *Shrek.*

    b. *Rambo.*

    c. *Star Wars.*

    d. *Life and Depth.*

89. Caring clowns are

    a. circus clowns who make hospital visits.

    b. clowns who work in all areas of health care.

    c. always professional actors.

    d. clowns who work only with children.

90. Eloise Cole (Rainbow) uses her clown character to help people who are

    a. bereaved.

    b. mentally ill.

    c. children.

    d. elderly.

91. The best way to become a Caring Clown is to

    a. attend training at a clown school.

    b. just have the desire to be funny.

    c. go with your natural instincts.

    d. be sure you have a gimmick.

92. A recommended guideline for Caring Clowns to follow during visitations is

    a. stay in the room as long as the patient wants.

    b. always give the patient something to remember you by.

    c. ask the patient for permission to enter the room.

    d. every visit should be made with a nurse present in the room.

93. When considering starting a humor program in a facility, the *most* appropriate way of helping administration *understand the benefits* of a humor program would be to

    a. present research information about the benefits of humor.

    b. have a clown come to the facility in costume to 'clown' with the administration.

    c. give them some articles to read about humor programs.

    d. immediately start a program to prove how successful it can be.

CHAPTER 13

HUMOR RX FOR YOUR PRACTICE

CHAPTER OBJECTIVES

After completing this chapter, the reader will be able to discuss ways to engage in humorous interchanges with patients, colleagues, and other healthcare providers.

LEARNING OBJECTIVES

After studying this chapter, the reader will be able to

1. discuss ways to bring humor into his or her own life.

2. identify appropriate humor.

3. recognize when it is inappropriate to use humor with a patient.

4. discuss ways to add more humor into the work environment.

INTRODUCTION

Medicine has many amusing occupational hazards.

— *Joel Goodman*

This chapter looks at interventions that can add humor into your practice. Working with patients or clients who are ill or having difficulty coping can add stress to those caring for them. Humor helps care providers to survive and deal with the stressors of administering health care. This chapter discusses ways to increase humor during patient care as well as ways to use humor with colleagues and other healthcare team members. Suggestions for improving or increasing personal humor experiences are also shared.

FOR YOURSELF

To bring humor into the healthcare environment, a sense of playfulness is helpful. As noted in the theory section of this course, playfulness is an essential component of humor. It helps us lighten up. It does what Joel Goodman of the Humor Project tells his audience to do: It lets you put the "elf" in "yourself" Until you find the humor within you, it can be hard to share humor with others. The following list suggests ways to add more humor into your life including some real-life examples:

- Watch funny movies.
- Watch sitcoms or comedy channels.
- Find the funny things in everyday situations.
  - A woman with dementia was cold, so she turned up the thermostat. Her husband became upset that she did this, so he turned the thermostat down and the air conditioner came on. It eventually became very cold in the house. The woman's daughter-in-law was using the telephone; her son and husband were watching television. Suddenly, the woman, who used to be very prim and proper, came out of the bedroom dressed in

her underwear and trying to put on her robe. The only problem was that she was trying to put her foot into the sleeve of the robe. Although this was really sad to see, the daughter-in-law could not help smiling at the ridiculous sight and the apparent oblivion of the woman's husband and son – neither of whom got up to help until the daughter-in-law stopped her conversation on the phone long enough to say, "Someone please help Mom."

– A student is at a library checking out some books. The student hands her card to the library assistant. The assistant looks at the card and says, "Oh, you've expired." The student looks around, looks back at the assistant, and says, "I don't think so."

– You are sitting in a gynecologist's office filling out a form. You get to a question that reads, "Are you presently sexually active?" Mind you, you are sitting in the doctor's waiting room. You think that there should be a box for "Not right at this moment."

- Think about and share an embarrassing story.

  – A lady went into a store dressing room to try on some bathing suits. As she went to put her leg into the leg of one suit, she lost her balance and fell out of the dressing room, in clear view of everyone standing outside the room.

  – A woman was walking down a busy city street with her husband and a male friend. Suddenly a car stopped and a woman said to the lady, "Excuse me honey, but your skirt is caught in your pantyhose." And neither one of the men had noticed.

  – Many years ago, a candy striper who was very short was preparing to throw laundry down the laundry shoot. The laundry cart was very tall. As she reached in to get the laundry, she fell into the laundry basket.

There she was with her feet in the air and her head in the cart. The head nurse walked by and said, "Okay, Nancy, get yourself out of there." Eventually, they had to obtain help to get her out.

- Keep a humor log or journal of jokes, experiences, puns, cartoons, and stories that made you laugh each day.

  – A woman who had a bad skin condition kept a humor diary as a way of improving her sense of humor. The more humor she found, the more she began to enjoy things around her, and the better her skin condition became.

- Blow bubbles

  – Pens that have bubbles on one end make great items to carry with you. One day, a 3-year-old was crying and acting up in the airport. Out came the bubbles. For 15 minutes, the child stopped crying and the grown-ups smiled. The atmosphere became less tense.

- Collect stress-releasing toys. Examples of great toys are clown noses, Groucho glasses, and toys that make animal noises or growl.

  – Clown noses work great in traffic. One "jollyologist" likes to put on a red clown nose and watch all the people around him when they notice it.

  – One lady with cancer received a toy that looked like a funny face. When she squeezed it, the eyes and tongue popped out. Whenever she was feeling stressed, she would pull out the face and squeeze it.

  – A counseling student was doing her internship at a community college. One of the counselors had just lost her husband and was having a number of difficult days. Plus, it was the beginning of registration and the tension level was high. One day, the student brought in a stuffed dinosaur that growled when it was squeezed. The toy was such a big hit with the counselor that she bought the counselor a baby dinosaur that did not have as loud of a roar. One day, the student heard the growl of the baby dinosaur many times. Thinking the counselor was having a bad day, she stopped in to say hello and found a member of the office staff there instead. The office worker explained that she was going through a really difficult time and the growl of the baby dinosaur brought a smile to her face.

- Collect toys when you see them. For example, a few years ago, a discount store was selling a little box that looked like a shipping box. At one corner, it looked as if an eye was peeking out. If you pushed the button on the other corner, the box would shake and a little voice could be heard: "Help! Help! Somebody let me out of here."

- Watch children at play.

- Play with children.

- Watch the antics of animals.

- Take silly photos of yourself making funny faces or doing something silly. Keep the photos where you will look at them to remind yourself to maintain a playful attitude.

- Make a list of things that you have fun doing and do two of them each day.

- Place reminders to take time for play in key areas (such as on a bathroom mirror, refrigerator, or desk).

- Hang around people who have positive attitudes and make you laugh. When you are around negative people, they bring you down. Find people who find enjoyment in life and can laugh at the everyday annoyances. When you are with others who are playful and help you laugh, you add that much more humor to your life.

- Make up a humor "first-aid kit" containing items that make you laugh. The kit might con-

tain such items as funny cartoons, cards, bumper stickers, bouncing balls, whistles, or funny hats. When you or someone you know is down, pull out something from the kit.

- Make a list of five things that make you smile. Then try to find five new things every day.

- Use exaggeration. Take a bad day at work and really blow it out of proportion. The more exaggeration, the better. Eventually, the humor in the situation is likely to come out. Share it with co-workers and have them add to the exaggeration.

- Smile, even if you do not feel like it. Your face does not know the difference between the real thing and a forced smile, and it can help lighten your mood. Also, others will wonder what you are up to!

- Do something you do not normally do. Doing or saying something unexpected causes you and others to pause and usually results in a smile or even a laugh.

  - Rather than answer "I'm fine" when someone asks how you are, say something like, "It depends on who you ask, but I think I'm great!"

  - One humor presenter shared how, occasionally, at a toll booth he would pay for the car behind him, and then watch the surprised and quizzical expressions on the faces of the people in the car as they tried to figure out what happened and why.

- Declare a funny hat day at work. (Obtain administration's permission first.) It is fun for the staff as well as for the patients.

- Wear or carry something humorous.

  - A lady at a local bagel shop wears a different headpiece every day. She has a headband with springs to which she attaches items. Some days it has windmills on it, other days it has hearts that wiggle or multicolored balls.

- Find a pen that is different, such as one that looks like a syringe or one that holds bubble soap and a wand.

• Laugh at life's daily slip-ups.

- When you put the cereal in the refrigerator or the milk in the cabinet, laugh about it.

• Laugh it up. A hearty belly laugh may be better for you than a demure giggle.

• Stay alert for humor on the job

- A social worker was talking to a patient whose family member had just had surgery. After a lengthy talk about what the patient is going to need after she gets out of surgery, the social worker asked, "Are you the closest relative?" The family member quickly responded, "Oh no, I live clear over in Virginia."

- An elderly man with mild dementia came into the emergency room. The person taking his admissions information asked him what brought him to the hospital. He looked at her quizzically and said, "Why, the taxi."

HUMOR AND PATIENT CARE

We know that using humor with patients is a way of establishing rapport, communicating in a nonthreatening manner, enhancing teaching opportunities, and decreasing stress and anxiety. Humor may be initiated by the patient or the healthcare provider. In some situations, such as crises, the health professional commonly waits for the patient to be the initiator. If the provider chooses to be the initiator, it is best to follow the advice of Karyn Buxman (1996; Gross, Buxman & Ayers, 2009): Be sure you follow the "Five Rights of Humor Administration."

The type of humor that is most often a part of the interaction between patient and provider is situational humor. It occurs spontaneously and reflects the present situation between healthcare personnel and patient. This type of humor can offer a sense of control in a powerless situation. As Klein (n.d.) states, "Laughter is a powerful tool in a powerless situation" (p. 5). It can offer hope and an upper hand to patients who are experiencing physical and mental loss. Allen Klein (n.d.) offers sound advice when it comes to using humor:

> The safest way…is to first establish a rapport with the patient. Then look for humor by listening to what the patient jokes about. Above all, do not go into a patient's room with a battery of jokes. First, jokes can be offensive, and second, when you enter the room of someone who is ill, you have no knowledge whether they will be receptive to your kidding around (p. 6).

Paying attention to the words used to create the humor can give the healthcare provider clues about the type of humor a patient is comfortable with. Humor can also cover up issues that may need to be explored. For this reason, providers need to think of humor as a therapeutic clue from which to build. For example, a dying patient says to a provider, "I wish we had pop-up buttons like turkeys, so we'd know when we were done!" (Robinson, 1991, p. 52). The message here has something to do with the anxiety of waiting to die. An alert provider can use this statement to open up communication regarding the patient's concern.

Culture, personality, level of stress, pain, and depression are all factors that need to be considered when initiating or responding to humor with patients. Initiating humor with terminally ill patients requires sensitivity. Terminally ill participants of a study by Herth (1995) suggested that attempts at humor by healthcare providers should begin slowly using lighthearted responses, such as smiling, winking, or playful comments (Herth,

> A motorcycle patrolman was rushed to the hospital with an inflamed appendix. The doctors operated and advised him that all was well. However, the patrolman kept feeling something pulling at the hairs on his chest.
>
> Worried that it might be a second surgery the doctors hadn't told him about, he finally got enough energy to pull his hospital gown down enough so he could look at what was making him so uncomfortable.
>
> Taped firmly across his hairy chest were three wide strips of adhesive tape, the kind that doesn't come off easily.
>
> Written in large black letters was the sentence:
>
> "Get well quick, from the nurse you gave a ticket to last week."
>
> *Note.* From NursingHumor.com. Used with permission.

1995). "Openness to fun on the clinician's part can provide the opportunity for the seriously ill individual to open up to humor" (Herth, 1995, p. 224).

A gentleman in the hospital had asked his wife to bring in some of his toys. One of them was a toy that made the sound of glass crashing when you hit the bottom of it. It was not uncommon for members of the staff to come in and borrow his toys to cause smiles and laughter in the life of other patients. Plus, the doctors would start their rounds by playing with his toys. It delighted him to be able to provide that type of entertainment for others, and the staff knew it. The toys also gave staff permission to joke with him. Supporting the use of toys is one of the ways healthcare providers can help support and encourage humor use by patients.

Prior to initiating humor with a patient, it is helpful to know what that particular patient finds funny. A formal method of doing this would be to use the humor assessment offered in chapter 4. A full assessment may not always be needed. Ask one assessment question and build on it. For example: "What is your favorite sitcom?" When the patient

answers, respond with, "What is it about the program that you like?" As the discussion progresses, ask the patient to share a favorite scene. As the patient shares, note if the patient's mood lightens. It probably will. After all, who can recall the Lucille Ball scene where she is stomping on the grapes and not begin to at least smile?

Above all else, smile whenever and wherever appropriate. The connection between healthcare provider and patient, or healthcare provider and visitor, grows from the smile. Stay alert to the patient's use of humor, and look for times when humor can be interjected. Just remember the Five Rights and remain alert for the right as well as the wrong time.

Personal Insight

During the development of my dissertation, I found that simply asking about participants' use of humor in coping with breast cancer increased their awareness of how they use humor in their lives. The result for a number of participants was to deliberately increase and be aware of humor in their lives. So, a simple question might be, "What role has humor had in your life?" Approaching the subject, giving the patient permission to think about and pursue humor, is a simple intervention that can help lead the patient to moments of coping humor.

Add humor to your patient education. Remember that humor catches the imagination, can decrease tension, and may increase learning. Be alert to the patient's use of humor as a message of concern, and use that as a means of leading into teaching situations. Caring requires that healthcare providers be alert for opportunities to teach patients the way to better health, be it for prevention or for managing a disease process. Smile; it helps the patient feel more at ease, and decreased tension leads to increased retention of information.

THE WRONG TIME, THE WRONG TYPE

There are times when humor is not appropriate. For humor to be effective, healthcare providers must be alert for the right time to use it. At times, humor can be hurtful and even detrimental. As mentioned in chapter 7, the survivor of a disaster or crisis might initiate humor, but initiation by the provider during the immediate crisis situation is often inappropriate.

In some cases, what the patient needs to do is cry or yell, or be quiet and alone. Watch for those times. Encourage patients to do what they need to do at that time. Sometimes just saying the right words at the right time is what a patient needs. Sometimes what a patient needs to hear is "this stinks" or "this sucks."

The wrong type of humor can cause discomfort or even anger. Avoid joking that pokes fun at other individuals or groups, such as cultural or political jokes. Using put-downs, ethnic jokes; "anti-" jokes (jokes that are negative toward men, women, religious or ethnic groups) are usually hurtful. Sarcasm and gallows humor can also be hurtful. The safest form of humor is self-effacing humor. Just remember to make fun of what you do, not who you are.

HUMOR INTERVENTIONS FOR SURVIVING WORK-INDUCED STRESS

A very good bit of advice when work is stress-filled is to take your work seriously and yourself lightly. Burnout, or "compassion fatigue" as it has been called, is a hazard anyone in a helping profession faces. During times of burnout, humor can be hard to find. However, if we can manage to tap into our funny bone, laughter and play change thinking and attitudes and can do a lot to prevent or decrease the sense of apathy that burnout can cause.

There are many stressors within the healthcare environment. When staff members are stressed, overworked, and out of sorts, it is a good idea to bring some humor into the environment. Things that staff can do for themselves include sharing cartoons on bulletin boards, taking funny photos and sharing them, telling jokes, supporting and applauding efforts of staff members, giving each other a standing ovation, and wearing a humorous item to work.

This is the story of what one person did to lighten her mood and get her point across:

The head nurse had left her job and one of the staff nurses was assigned to be "schedule coordinator." Everyone on the floor did his or her own scheduling, but she was the overseer who checked for over- or understaffing, and made appropriate changes. She made enemies in the process. After a few months of hate mail, she posted the following message.

"Following the path of our Congressmen and Senators, I am pleased to inform you I will now be accepting bribes. Twenty dollars per request, regular weekday. Twenty-five dollars per holiday or weekend request. Guaranteed fulfillment of your request! The money will go to my Special Defense Fund. I've hired a bodyguard to protect me from the wrath of all of you!"

As a gift for having endured this test, here are some one-liners you might be able to use:

- A clean desk is a sign of a cluttered desk drawer.

- A flashlight is a case for holding dead batteries.

- All generalizations are false, including this one.

- Always remember you're unique, just like everyone else.

- Be nice to your kids. They'll choose your nursing home.

- Before you criticize someone, you should walk a mile in their shoes. That way, when you criticize them, you're a mile away and you have their shoes.

- Bills travel through the mail at twice the speed of checks.

- Consciousness: That annoying time between naps.

- Plan to be spontaneous, tomorrow.

- Smile! It increases your face value.

Discussion Questions

Rather than present a case study for this chapter, it was decided to pose some questions for you to think about. If this was a face-to-face class, these might be good discussion questions. So think about these, share them with your coworkers and look at how you might bring humor into the area you work to benefit your patients, yourself, and your coworkers.

1. What can you do to add more humor into your life?

2. What can you do in your work area to share your humor knowledge with others?

3. What steps can you take to bring humor into the lives of your patients/clients?

SUMMARY

Sometimes humor happens spontaneously and works as a means of connection between the healthcare provider and patient or the healthcare provider and another healthcare provider. Either way, it's helpful for healthcare providers to practice putting more humor into their lives to increase the likelihood of using humor more often with patients and coworkers. Some techniques for increasing the amount of humor in your life involve creating a more light-hearted environment through the addition of playful toys and tools. Some strategies include practicing behaviors such as journaling, joke telling or story telling. Other techniques involve looking within; play-

ing with your own mindset and perspective. Despite the fact that humor can be therapeutic, there are times when humor is appropriate, and times when it is not. There are also certain types of humor that do not have a place in the healthcare setting. Bottom line: Be sensitive to others and honor your ability to find funny things in everyday experiences.

Lessons from the chapter:

- To add humor into the workplace to help your patients, you must first have humor in your life.
  - Be alert to ways of adding humor.
  - Remember to take yourself lightly while you take your work seriously.

- When putting humor in patient care
  - be sensitive.
  - be alert.
  - develop rapport.
  - look for opportunities to lighten the tension.
  - smile, it makes you feel better, and helps those around you.

- Types of humor to avoid:
  - Put-down, sarcastic humor
  - Ethnic jokes
  - Anti-jokes
  - Gallows or black humor
    - It might be appropriate with coworkers, but it is not appropriate with patients.

- Be sure it is the right time. Patients and staff need to be emotionally receptive to humor and there are times when humor is just not appropriate.

- Interventions to prevent "compassion fatigue."
  - Although it is important to take your work seriously, take yourself lightly.
  - Look for the funny side of life.

EXAM QUESTIONS

CHAPTER 13
Questions 94-100

Note: Choose the one option that BEST answers each question.

94. You are late for work. Traffic is backed up and barely moving because of an accident. Something needs to be done to break your tension and the tension of the drivers around you. Taking the advice of this text, you

    a. start screaming.
    b. close your eyes and hope the other drivers will wake you up.
    c. put on a clown nose.
    d. take out a magazine and start reading.

95. The Five Rights of Humor Administration are

    a. right patient, right trigger, right time, right amount, right route.
    b. right patient, right type, right focus, right amount, right route.
    c. right patient, right type, right time, right amount, right cue.
    d. right patient, right type, right time, right amount, right route.

96. The most common type of humor between patient and nurse is

    a. situational.
    b. planned.
    c. programmed.
    d. joking.

97. A patient has been admitted with a diagnosis of congestive heart failure. The nurse is concerned about the patient's sad mood and decides that humor might be appropriate. Taking the advice of Allen Klein, she decides to

    a. go into the room with a few jokes she can share.
    b. wear a clown nose when entering the room.
    c. bring a book of The Far Side jokes with her into the room.
    d. establish rapport and listen for clues from the patient.

98. The type of humor that should be avoided by the nurse is

    a. work-related humor.
    b. puns.
    c. anti-jokes.
    d. situational humor.

99. One way to help prevent compassion fatigue is to

    a. find ways to play.
    b. share your complaints with others.
    c. become politically active.
    d. put in more hours at work.

continued on next page

100. Tensions were rising on the medical unit. One of the nurses decided to add some humor to try and decrease the tension. He wanted to do something that all might be able to enjoy. The best way for him to do this is to

   a.   share cartoons pertaining to healthcare mishaps.

   b.   share ethnic jokes with the staff.

   c.   play practical jokes on his coworkers.

   d.   bring comedy videos for the staff to watch.

This concludes the final examination.

Please answer the evaluation questions found on page v of this workbook.

RESOURCES

Web Resources

Allen Klein, The Jollyologist

Allen Klein is an award-winning professional speaker and best-selling author of such books as *The Healing Power of Humor, The Courage to Laugh,* and *Up Words for Down Days.* His Web site contains humor-related articles, links to other humor sites, and a listing of recommended humor books.
http://www.allenklein.com/

Art Gliner Center for Humor Studies

This center offers a scholarship for graduate student internship proposals to work on training that will lead to socially useful applications of humor. There is a link to essays on humor as well as other humor sites.
http://www.humorcenter.umd.edu

Association for Applied and Therapeutic Humor (AATH)

This is a great Web site that contains articles, general information on therapeutic and applied humor, and information on conferences. AATH is an international community of professionals who incorporate humor in their lives and practices; they provide evidence-based information about current research and practical applications of humor.
http://www.aath.org/

Good Humor, Good Health

This site has an article written by David S. Sobel, MD, MPH, and Robert Ornstein, PhD, that discusses how humor can be used to stay healthy.
http://www.kaiserpermanente.org/toyourhealth/hottopics/sobel/humor.html

How Laughter Works

This article, from the How Stuff Works Web site, looks at what happens in our brains when we laugh, what makes us laugh, and how laughter can make us healthier and happier. The article ends with tips for putting more laughter into our lives and links to other useful Web sites.
http://www.howstuffworks.com/laughter

Humor for Your Health

This Canadian organization was launched to empower people to obtain greater health and happiness through the understanding and application of their own unique sense of humor. The site has articles on the ancient history of humor and health, using humor at work and at school, the keys to telling jokes, surviving grief with humor, appropriate and inappropriate humor, and much more!
http://humorforyourhealth.com

Humor Matters

Presented by Dr. Steven Sultanoff, former President of the Association for Applied and Therapeutic Humor, this Web site is dedicated to educate, inform, and help visitors network and locate resources that focus on humor and its relation to health and healing.
http://humormatters.com

Humor Research

This page has great links to information about humor research, humor researchers, Web pages, where many of the researchers offer information about the research they have done, and a list of courses being taught about humor. http://www.uni-duesseldorf.de/ WWW/MathNat/Ruch/humor.html

International Society for Humor Studies

The purpose of the International Society for Humor Studies is to encourage and share humor research studies in all areas of academics. This site provides connections to articles, information on conferences, a series of bibliographies, a list of members involved in humor research and humor studies links. http://www.hnu.edu/ishs/index.htm

Jest for the Health of It!

Patty Wooten has put together this great Web site for information on humor; buying humor books, tapes, or other products; therapeutic clowning; and humor links. http://www.jesthealth.com

Journal of Nursing Jocularity

The only humor magazine by and for nurses. Contains entertainment and educational pieces on the application of humor for patient care, self-care, education, and more. www.JournalOfNursingJocularity.com

Laryngospasms. A group of four nurse anesthetists who combine their medical background with their sense of humor and singing talents to create and perform medical parodies of classic and familiar songs. www.laryngospasms.com

Laughter Remedy

This Web site was created by Paul McGhee. There is information about the health benefits of humor as well as how individuals, organizations and support groups can benefit from humor. http://www.laughterremedy.com

Laughter Yoga International

An international organization dedicated to therapeutic laughter, founded by Madan Kataria. Information on therapeutic laughter, trainings, events, and more. http://www.laughteryoga.org/

Managed Music

A musical group led by Dr. Sam Bierstock, primarily blues in nature. They address various health care topics. www.managedmusic.com

NurseTogether.com

A nurse community Web site that includes a wide variety of resources, articles, forums, media and more for nurses on topics related to stress management, life balance, humor, and more. www.NurseTogether.com

NurSING Notes.

A barbershop quartet of nurses spreading healthcare humor through harmony. www.thenursingnotes.com

NursTOON.com.

An online resource for nursing cartoons. www.nursetoons.com

Nursing & Medical Humor links on:

The Nurse Friendly

This site offers humorous stories and nursing jokes as well as information on travel nursing, home businesses, and other general information.
http://www.nursinghumor.com

Rx Laughter

This site provides information on the study of laughter in children.
http://www.rxlaughter.org/

The Humor Collection

This page offers links to other humor pages, humor information, information on humor research, and more.
http://www.thehumorcollection.org

The Humor Project

The Humor Project was started by Joel Goodman in Sarasota, New York. This Web site offers information about the project, humor discussion boards, materials for purchase, conference information, and more.
http://www.humorproject.com/

Standup for Mental Health

Mental health consumers turn their problems into comedy, then perform their acts at conferences, treatment centers, psych wards, for various mental health organizations, on college and university campuses, and general public. Great examples of applied and therapeutic humor in mental health.
http://www.standupformentalhealth.com/

The Magic Corner

This site has an online catalog of magic supplies, clowning accessories, and juggling equipment. There is also information about classes and events.
http://www.themagiccorner.com/

Too Live Nurse.

A musical group providing education through music and humor for healthcare professionals.
www.toolivenurse.com

Twitter.com/FunnyNurse

Brief posts related to nursing humor. All posts are 140 characters or less. Many contain links to additional Web sites or resources.
www.Twitter.com/FunnyNurse

World Laughter Tour

This is the official page for the World Laughter Tour. There is information about Laughter Clubs, becoming a certified laughter leader, as well as articles discussing laughter and its contribution to health.
http://www.worldlaughtertour.com

REFERENCES

A Prairie Home Companion Pretty Good Joke Book. (2005). Minneapolis: Highbridge Company.

Abel, M.H. (1998). Interaction of humor and gender in moderating relationships between stress and outcomes. *Journal of Psychology, 132*(3), 267-276. Retrieved January 25, 2009, from http://epnet.com

Adamle, K.N. (2001). *Social interaction in hospice work: A study of humor.* Dissertation, Kent State. Retrieved January 25, 2009, from ProQuest Dissertations.

Adams, H. (1993). Humor: Strong medicine. *International Journal of Arts Medicine,* (2)3. Retrieved December 1, 2008, from EbscoHost.

Adams, P. (2002). Humour and love: The origination of clown therapy. *Postgraduate Medical Journal, 78*(922), 447-478(2). Retrieved January 25, 2009, from http://pmj.bmj.com/cgi/content/full/78/922/447

Allnurses.com (nd) *Fallopian tube!!!* Retrieved May 10, 2009 from http://allnurses.com/nursing-humor-share/fallopian-tube-259529.html

Astedt-Kurki, P. & Isola, A. (2001). Humour between nurse and patient, and among staff: Analysis of nurses' diaries. *Journal of Advanced Nursing, 35*(3), 452-458.

Association for Applied and Therapeutic Humor. (n.d.) Retrieved February 5, 2009, from http://www.aath.org

Bachorowski, J. & Owren, M. (2004, September). Laughing matters. *Science Briefs, 18*(9), 1-5. Retrieved November 20, 2008, from http://www.apa.org/science/psa/sb-bachprt.html

Baldwin, E. (2007). Humor perception: The contribution of cognitive factors. (UMI Number 3278576). Retrieved May 3, 2008, from UMI ProQuest Digital Dissertations.

Balick, M.J. & Lee, R. (2003) *The Role of Laughter in Traditional Medicine and its Relevance to the Clinical Setting: Healing with HA! Alternative Therapies,* July/Aug. 2003, Vol. 9, N. 4. Retrieved June 2, 2010, from http://sciweb.nybg.org/Science2/pdfs/mb/august.pdf

Bandura, A. (1997, March). Self-efficacy. *Harvard Mental Health Letter 13*(9). Retrieved January 25, 2009, from Academic Search Premier database.

Barasch, D.S. (1999, March). Sense of humor. *Family Life,* 40-42.

Bariaud, F. (1989). Age differences in children's humor. In P.E. McGhee (Ed.), *Humor and children's development: A guide to practical applications* (pp. 15-45). New York: Haworth Press.

Bartlett, T. (2003). Did you hear the one about the professor? *Chronicle of Higher Education, 49*(46, A8-A10. Retrieved January 25, 2009, from EBSCO Host database.

Bauer, M.E., Gauer, G.J., Luz, C., Silveira, R.O., Nardi, N.B., & von Muhlen, C.A. (1995). Evaluation of immune parameters in depressed patients. *Life Sciences, 57*(7), 655-674.

Bazzini, D.G., Stack, E.R., Martincin, P.D., & Davis, C.P. (2006). The effect of reminiscing about laughter on relationship satisfaction. *Motivation Emotion, 31,* 25-34.

Baycrest Centre for Geriatric Care. (2003, August 25). *Appreciation of humor doesn't change with age.* Retrieved January 25, 2009, from http://www.baycrest.org/News_and_Media/News_Releases_2003/default_6611.asp

Beck, C.T. (1997). Humor in nursing practice: A phenomenological study. *International Journal of Nursing Studies, 34*(5), 346-352.

Bellert, J. (1989). Humor: A therapeutic approach in oncology nursing. *Cancer Nursing, 12*(2), 65-70.

Bennett, M.P., Zeller, J.M., Rosenberg, L., & McCann, J. (2003). The effect of mirthful laughter on stress and natural killer cell activity. *Alternative Therapies in Health and Medicine, 9*(2), 38-45.

Berger, A.A. (1987). Humor: An introduction. *American Behavioral Scientist, 30*(1), 6-15.

Berk, L.S., Felten, D.L., Tan, S.A., Bittman, B.B., & Westengard, J. (2001). Modulation of neuro-immune parameters during the eustress of humor-associated mirthful laughter. *Alternative Therapies in Health and Medicine, 7*(2), 62-76.

Berk, L.S., Tan, S.A., Fry, W.F., Napier, B.J., Lee, J.W., Hubbard, R.W., et al. (1989, December). Neuroendocrine and stress hormone changes during mirthful laughter. *American Journal of the Medical Sciences, 298*(6), 390-396.

Berk, R.A. (2002). *Humor as an instructional defibrillator: Evidence-based: Techniques in teaching and assessment.* Sterling, VA: Stylus Publishing.

Bhosai, S.J., Miwa, S., Hilber, S.D. (2007) Understanding the effects of humor therapy on the patient's self-reports of pain, comfort, and anxiety. Rx Laughter & NCI Thailand. Retrieved December 7, 2008, from http://www.rxlaughter.org/RxLNCIfinalApril2nd2007.doc

Bihn, P. (1995). Starting a humor cart. *Journal of Nursing Jocularity, 5*(2), 32-34.

Bippus, A.M. (2000). Humor usage in comforting episodes: Factors predicting outcomes. *Western Journal of Communication, 64*(4), 359-384.

Boerman-Cornell, W. (2000). "Humor" your students! *Education Digest, 5*(65), 56-62. Retrieved January 25, 2009, from EBSCO Host database.

Bokun, B. (1986). *Humour therapy in cancer, psychosomatic diseases, mental disorders, crime, interpersonal and sexual relationships.* London: Vita Books.

Bottari, A.C. (2000). Humor in Healing. *Subconsciously Speaking, 15*(6). Retrieved February 20, 2009, from EBSCO Host database.

Bower, G.H. & Hilgard, E.R. (1981). *Theories of Learning.* Englewood Cliffs, NJ: Prentice-Hall.

Brilliantt, A. (1981). *Appreciate me now and avoid the rush.* Santa Barbara, CA: Woodbridge Press.

Brookfield, S.D. (1986). *Understanding and facilitating adult learning: A comprehensive analysis of principles and effective practices.* San Francisco: Jossey-Bass.

Buxman, K. (1991). Make room for laughter. *American Journal of Nursing, 91*(12), 46-51.

Buxman, K. (1996). 5 rights of humor administration. Presented at the Journal of Nursing Jocularity Humor Skills for the Health Professional Conference, St. Louis, MO.

Buxman, K. (1998). *Humor as a cost-effective means of stress management.* Retrieved May 9, 2009, from http://www.karynbuxman.com/2009/05/15/humor-as-a-cost-effective-means-of-stress-management

Buxman, K. (2000). Humor in critical care: No joke. *AACN Clinical Issues, 11*(1), 120-127.

Buxman, K. (2000). *This won't hurt a bit! And other fractured truths in healthcare.* Hannibal, MO: LaMoine Press.

Buxman, K. (2001). *Mind if I laugh? Humor when tragedy strikes.* Retrieved May 9, 2009, from http://www.karynbuxman.com/2008/09/01/mind-if-i-laugh-humor-when-tragedy strikes

Buxman, K. (2008). Humor in the OR: A stitch in time? *AORN Journal, 1*(88), 67-77.

Canfield, J, Hansen, M.V., Mitchell-Autio, N., & Thieman, L. (2001) *Chicken Soup for the Nurse's Soul: 101 Stories to Celebrate, Honor and Inspire the Nursing Profession.* Health Communications Inc., Dearfield Beach. FL.

Carver, C.S., Pozo, C., Harris, S.D., Noriega, V., Scheier, M.F., Robinson, D.S., et al. (1993). How coping mediates the effect of optimism on distress: A study of women with early stage breast cancer. *Journal of Personality and Social Psychology, 65*(2), 375-390.

Cheagn, H.S. & Pell, M.D. (2006). A study of humour and communicative intention following right hemisphere stroke. *Clinical Linguistics & Phonetics, 20*(6), 447-462.

Clark, W.N. (2002). What makes babies laugh? *Parenting, 16*(7), 191-192. Retrieved March 1, 2009, from EBSCO Host database.

Coffee, G. (1990). *Beyond survival: Building on the hard times – A POW's inspiring story.* New York: Putnam.

Cole, E. (2001). *Humor and grief.* Paper presented at the American Association for Therapeutic Humor Annual Conference, February 2-4, 2001.

Conkell, C., Imwold, C., & Ratliffe, T. (1999). The effects of humor on communicating fitness concepts to high school students. *Physical Educator, 56*(1). Retrieved February 20, 2009, from EBSCO Host database.

Cousins, N. (1979). *Anatomy of an illness as perceived by the patient: Reflections on healing and regeration.* New York: Bantam.

Cundall, M.K. (2007) Humor and the limits of incongruity. *Creativity Research Journal, 19*(2-3), 203-211.

Darby, M. (1996). *Humor and the treatment of mental illness: Use it or lose it!* Omaha, NE: Surprise Publishing.

Doskoch, P. (1996). Happily ever laughter. *Psychology Today, 29*(4), 32-36.

Dossey, L. (1996). "Now you are fit to live": Humor and health. *Alternative Therapies in Health and Medicine, 2*(5), 8-13. Retrieved March 1, 2009, from EBSCO Host database.

Dowling, J.S. (2002). Humor: A coping strategy for pediatric patients. *Pediatric Nursing, 28*(2), 123-131.

Driver, J.L. & Gottman, J.M. (2004) Daily marital interactions and positive affect during marital conflict among newlywed couples. *Family Process, 3*(43), 301-314.

Dworetzky, J.P. & Davis, N.J. (1989). *Human development: A lifespan approach.* St. Paul: West Publishing.

Elderhostel (n.d.). *About Elderhostel.* Retrieved February 18, 2009, from http://www.elderhostel.org/about/default.asp

Elias, M. (2003). Happy folks live longer than fuddy-duddies. *USA Today.* Retrieved February 14, 2009, from http://www.usatoday.com/news/health/2003-03-04-happy_x.htm

Ferraro, K.F. (Ed.) (1997). *Gerontology: Perspectives and issues* (2nd ed.). New York: Springer.

Flatter, C. (1995.). Two to five year olds. In *A look at humor in children through the years.* Sesame Street Supplement Issue, 248, p78-80.

Fletcher, D. (1991). Editor's note. *Journal of Nursing Jocularity, 1*(4), 3.

Flournoy, E., Turner, G., & Combs, D. (2001). Read the writing on the wall. *Nursing2001, 31*(3), 32cc8-32cc10.

Flowers, J. (2001, May/June). The value of humor in technology education. *The Technology Teacher,* 10-12.

Foltz-Gray, D. (1998). Make 'em laugh: Humor programs can help residents heal – seriously. *Contemporary Longterm Care, 21*(9), 44-46.

Ford-Martin, P. (2001). Stress. *Gale encyclopedia of alternative medicine.* Retrieved March 10, 2009, from http://findarticles.com/p/articles/mi_g 2603/is_0006/ai_2603000686?tag=content;col1

Frankl, V.E. (1963). *Man's search for meaning: An introduction to logotherapy.* New York: Simon & Shuster.

Frecknall, P. (1994). Good humor: A qualitative study of the uses of humor in everyday life. *Psychology: A Journal of Human Behavior, 31*(1), 12-21.

Freud, S. (1960). *Jokes and their relation to the unconscious* (J. Strachey, Trans.). New York: W.W. Norton. (Original work published 1905).

Fuhr, M. (2002). Coping humor in early adolescence. *Humor, 15*(3), 283-304.

Gascon, D. (1998). Illness is a laughing matter. *Humor for your health.* Retrieved March 5, 2009, from http://www.bradmontgomery.com/resources/about-humor-motivation-laughter/what-is-healing-humor

Gelkopf, M., Sigal, M., & Kramer, R. (1994). Therapeutic use of humor to improve social support in an institutionalized schizophrenic inpatient community. *The Journal of Social Psychology, 134*(2). Retrieved May 20, 2003, from InfoTrac.

Gervais, M. & Wilson, D.S. (2005). The evolution and functions of laughter and humor: A synthetic approach. *The Quarterly Review of Biology, 80,* 395-430.

Gibson, L. (1995). Comedy carts, baskets, and humor rooms. In K. Buxman & A. LeMoine (Eds.), *Nursing perspectives on humor.* Staten Island, NY: Power Publications.

Goldin, E. & Bordan, T. (1999, Fall). The use of humor in counseling: The laughing cure. *Journal of Counseling and Development, 77,* 405-410.

Goodboe, M.E. (1995, April). Should security practice andragogy? [Electronic version]. *Security Management, 39*(4).

Goodheart, A. (1994). *Laughter therapy: How to laugh about everything in your life that isn't really funny.* Santa Barbara, CA: Less Stress Press.

Gorfinkle, K.S., Slater, J.A., Bagiella, E., Tager, F.A., & Labinsky, E.B. (1998.). Child behavioral distress during invasive oncologic procedures and cardiac catheterization with the big apple circus clown care unit. *Pediatric Research: Volume, 43*(4) Supplement 2, April. Retrieved March 15, 2009, from http://www.journals.lww.com/pedresearch/Fulltext/1998/04001/Child_Behavioral_Distress_During_Invasive.76.aspx

Graves, P.L. (2008). When children tell stories: Developmental considerations. *Bulletin of the Menninger Clinic, 72*(1), 19-37.

Gross, S., Buxman, K., & Ayers, G. (2009). *The service prescription. Healthcare the way it was meant to be.* T. Scott Gross & Co. Inc, Kerrville, TX.

Groves, D.F. (1991). "A merry heart doeth good like a medicine…" *Holistic Nursing Practice, 5*(4), 49-56.

Grow, G. (1996, March 20). *Teaching learners to be self-directed.* Retrieved March 10, 2009, from http://www.longleaf.net/ggrow/SSDL/SSDLIndex.html

Gullickson, C. (1995). Listening beyond the laughter: Communicating through the use of humor. In K. Buxman & A. LeMoine (Eds.), *Nursing perspectives on humor.* Staten Island, NY: Power Publications.

Haig, R.A. (1988). *The anatomy of humor: Biopsychosocial and therapeutic perspectives.* Springfield, IL: Thomas.

Hamilton, R. (2003). *The joyful alternative.* Retrieved March 8, 2009, from http://www.rtpnetorg/~cahaha

Harvey, L.C. (1998). *Humor for healing: A therapeutic approach.* San Antonio, TX: Therapy Skill Builders.

Hayashi, K., Hayashi, T., Iwanaga, S., Kawai, K., Ishii, H., Shoji, S., et al. (2003). Laughter lowered the increase in postprandial blood glucose. *Diabetes Care, 265,* 1651-1652.

Henman, L.D. (2001). Humor as a coping mechanism: Lessons from POWs. *Humor, 14*(1), 83-94.

Hergenhahn, B.R. (1990). *An introduction to theories of personality* (3rd ed.). Englewood Cliffs, NJ: Prentice-Hall.

Herth, K.A. (1995). Humor's role in terminal illness. In K. Buxman & A. LeMoine (Eds.), *Nursing Perspectives on Humor.* Staten Island, NY: Power Publications.

Holland, N.N. (1982). *Laughing: A psychology of humor.* Ithaca, NY: Cornell University Press.

Howe, F.C. (1993). The child in elementary school. *Child Study Journal, 23*(4), 227-372.

Hudson, D. (2001). *Prescription for learning: Humor in the classroom.* Athens State University, Athens, AL. Retrieved March 7, 2009, from http://www.schoolmate.com/news/issues/fall01/fl01chalk.asp

Hugelshofer, D.S., Kwon, P., Reff, R.C., & Olson, M.L. (2006, March). Humour's role in the relation between attributional style and dysphoria. *European Journal of Personality, 20,* 325-336.

Huitt, W. (2001). Motivation to learn: An overview. *Educational Psychology Interactive.* Valdosta State University. Retrieved March 7, 2009, from http://www.edpsycinteractive.org/topics/motivation/motivate.html

Hunt, A.H. (1993). Humor as a nursing intervention. *Cancer Nursing, 16*(1), 34-39.

humor. (2009). In *Webster's New World College Dictionary.* Retrieved September 28th, 2009, from www.yourdictionary.com/humor

Humor in the brain: What happens when we laugh. An interview with Dr. Peter Derks (1995). *Humor & Health Letter, 4*(5).

Humor Matters. (n.d.). Definitions. Retrieved March 7, 2009, from http://www.humormatters.com/definiti.htm

Humor Project, Inc. (n.d.). *TimeLess: Humor-Wise and Humor Why's.* Retrieved June 10, 2010 from http://humorproject.com/about/humorwise.php

Isen, A.M., Daubman, K.A., & Nowicki, G.P. (1987). Positive affect facilitates creative problem solving. *Journal of Personality and Social Psychology, 52*(6), 1122-1131.

Jagetia, A., Kumar, N.P., Singh, D. & Sinha, S. (2006). Pathological laughter in trigeminal schwannoma: case report and review of the literature. *Neurosurgical Review, 29*(4), 348-352.

Jancin, B. (2001, March). Laughter benefits heart health, immune system. Retrieved March 7, 2009, from http://www.findarticles.com/p/articles/mi_m0BJI/is_6_31/ai_73181080

Johnson, P. (2002). The use of humor and its influences on spirituality and coping in breast cancer survivors. *Oncology Nursing Forum, 29*(4), 691-695.

Joshua, A.M., Cotroneo, A., & Clarke, S. (2005). Humor and oncology. *American Society of Clinical Oncology, 23*(3), 645-648.

Kaplan, R.M. & Pascoe, G.C. (1977). Humorous lectures and humorous examples: Some effects upon comprehension and retention. *Journal of Educational Psychology, 69*(1), 61-65.

Kaufman, G. (1991) *In stitches.* Bloomington, IN: Indiana University Press.

Kearsley, G. (1997, March 4). *Social learning theory. Exploration in learning & instruction: The theory into practice database.* Retrieved March 8, 2009, from http://tip.psychology.org/bandura.html

Kelly, L.Y. (1981). *Dimensions of professional nursing* (4th ed.). New York: MacMillan.

Kidd, M. (1990, September). Older women learning: Now and always [Electronic version]. *Women's Education-Education des femmes 8.* Retrieved March 8, 2009, from http://www.library.nald.cal/item/5328

Kiely, K. (2003, March 3). Vietnam POWs forged brotherhood in captivity. *USA Today.* Retrieved March 5, 2009, from www.aiipowmia.com/inter23/in030403brothers.html

Kinde, J. (2002). *Being funny on purpose: Developing original humor for your talk.* Retrieved March 10, 2009, from http://www.humorpower.com/original_humor.html

Kingsley, D. (2003, August #29). *Jokes not as funny as you get older.* Retrieved March 7, 2009, from http://www.abc.net.au/science/news/health/HealthRepublish_932837.htm

Klause, A.C. (1987, February). So what's so funny, anyway? *School Library Journal,* 34-35.

Kleiman, A.M. (1995, April 15). The aging agenda: Redefining library services for a graying population. *Library Journal, 120*(7), 32. Retrieved March 4, 2009, from EBSCO Host databank.

Klein, A. (n.d.). *Serious illness is not funny but funny things happen.* Retrieved March 8, 2009, from http://www.worldlaughtertour.com/pdfs/Allen_Klein_SERIOUS_ILLNESS_IS_NOT_FUNNY.pdf

Klein, A. (1989). *The healing power of humor.* Los Angeles: J.P. Tarcher.

Klein, A. (1992, Summer). Storybook humor and early development. *Childhood Education, 68*(4), 213-217.

Klein, A. (1998). *The courage to laugh: Humor, hope, and healing in the face of dying.* New York: J.P. Tarcher/Putnam.

Klein, A. (2001). How can you laugh at a time like this? *Association for Applied and Therapeutic Humor.* Retrieved March 9, 2009, from http://www.aath.org/articles/art_klein01.html

Klein, A.J. (1985). Humor comprehension and humor appreciation of cognitively oriented humor: A study of kindergarten children. *Child Study, 15*(4), 223-234.

Knight, B.G. (1996). *Psychotherapy with older adults* (2nd ed.). Thousand Oaks, CA: Sage Publications.

Knowles, M.S. (1978). *The adult learner: A neglected species.* Houston, TX: Gulf.

Kuhn, C. (2003). *The fun factor: Unleashing the power of humor at home and on the job* (2nd ed.). Louisville: Minerva Books.

Kuhn, C. (2006, December). *Healing with humor. Healthcare Financial Management.* Retrieved November 26, 2008, from http://findarticles. com/p/articles/mi_m3257/is_12_60/ai_n16911 303

Kuiper, N.A., Martin, R.A., & Olinger, L.J. (1993). Coping humor, stress, and cognitive appraisals. *Canadian Journal of Behavioral Science, 25*(1), 81-96.

Kutner, L. (n.d.). *Insights for parents: Humor as a key to child development.* Retrieved March 6, 2009, from http://www.drkutner.com/parenting/ articles/humor.html

Labott, S.M. & Martin, R.B. (1987, Winter). The stress-moderating effects of weeping and humor. *Journal of Human Stress, 13*(4), 159-164.

Labott, S.M., Ahleman, S., Wolever, M.E., & Martin, R.B. (1990, Winter). The physiological and psychological effects of the expression and inhibition of emotion. *Behavioral Medicine, 16*(4), 182-189.

Lamp, J.M. (1992). Humor in postpartum education: Depicting a new mother's worst nightmare. *Maternal-Child Nursing, 17*(2), 82-85.

Laughter Yoga International (n.d.) *Official Website of Dr. Kataria.* Retrieved February 18, 2009, from http://www.laughteryoga.org

Lawson, W. (2001). Engaging with humour. *Adults Learning, 12*(8). Retrieved March 5, 2009, from EBSCO Host databank.

Lebowitz, K.R. (2002). The effects of humor on cardiopulmonary functioning, psychological well-being, and health status among older adults with chronic obstructive pulmonary disease. (Publication Number: AAT 3049063). Retrieved March 8, 2009, from UMI ProQuest Digital Dissertations.

Lefcourt, H.M. & Martin, R.A. (1986). *Humor and life stress: Antidote to adversity.* New York: Springer-Verlag.

Lefcourt, H.M., Davidson, K., Shepherd, R., Phillips, M., Prakachin, K., & Mills, D. (1995). Perspective-taking humor: Accounting for stress moderation. *Journal of Social and Clinical Psychology, 14*(4), 373-391.

Leigh, E. (2001). *Triumph over tragedy.* Presented at the Association for Applied and Therapeutic Humor, 2001 workshop. San Diego, CA.

Leise, C.M. (1993). The correlation between humor and the chronic pain of arthritis. *Journal of Holistic Nursing, 11*(1), 82-95.

Le Vieux, J.S. (2002). *Use of humor in pediatric oncology patients as a coping mechanism: An ethnographic study.* (Doctoral dissertation). Retrieved from ProQuest Dissertations & Theses. (UMI No. 3059168).

Lippert, L.R. (2001). *Humor exchanges: An ethnographic study of humor as communication between nurses and residents in a long-term care residence* (Publication Number: AAT 3058609). Dissertation retrieved March 10, 2009, from ProQuest Dissertations.

Lomax, R.G. & Moosavi, S.A. (2002). Using humor to teach statistics: Must they be orthogonal? *Understanding Statistics, 1*(2), 113-130.

Long, H.B. (1990). Understanding adult learners. In M.W. Galbraith (Ed.), *Adult learning methods: A guide for effective instruction.* Malabar, FL: R.E. Krieger.

Love, S.M. (1991). *Dr. Susan Love's breast book.* New York: Addison-Wesley.

Lumsden, D.B. (1987-88, Winter). How adults learn. *Generations,* pp. 10-15.

Mahony, D.L. (2000). Is laughter the best medicine or any medicine at all? *Eye on Psi Chi, 4*(3), 18-21. Retrieved February 21, 2009, from http://www. psichi.org/pubs/articles/article_81.asp

Mahony, D.L., Burroughs, W.J., & Hieatt, A.C. (2001). The effects of laughter on discomfort thresholds: Does expectation become reality? *Journal of General Psychology, 128*(2), 217-226. Retrieved December 2, 2008, from EBSCO Host database.

Makinen, S., Suominen, T., & Lauri, S. (2000). Self-care in adults with asthma: How they cope. *Journal of Clinical Nursing, 9*(4), 557-565.

Malouf, D. (2003). *How to teach adults in a fun and exciting way* (2nd ed.). Crows Nest, NSW, Australia: Allen & Unwin.

Maranan, J.T. (2001, August). *Laughter may be a better antibiotic: Recent research proves that humor can help you fight germs.* Retrieved February 18, 2009, from http://www.find rticles.com/p/articles/mi_m0NAH/is_6_31/ai_ 80088276

Martin, R.A. & Lefcourt, H. (1983). Sense of humor as a moderator of the relation between stressors and moods. *Journal of Personality and Social Psychology, 45*(6), 1313-1324.

Martin, R.A. (1989). Humor and the mastery of living: Using humor to cope with the daily stresses of growing up. In P.E. McGhee (Ed.), *Humor and children's development: A guide to practical applications* (pp. 135-154). New York: Haworth Press.

Martin, R.A. (2001). Humor, laughter, and physical health: Methodological issues and research findings. *Psychological Bulletin, 127*(4), 504-519.

Martin, R.A. (2007). *The psychology of humor: An integrative approach.* San Diego: El Sevier.

Masie, E. (2003, March). Make it relevant, interesting …and funny. *ITTraining.* Retrieved March 4, 2009, from EBSCO Host database.

McCullough-Brabson, E. (1995, January). Teaching in the Elderhostel program. *Music Educators Journal, 8*(4), 41-44.

McGhee, P.E. (n.d.). *Humor and health.* Retrieved February 18, 2009, from http://www.holistic online.com/Humor_Therapy/humor_mcghee_ article.htm

McGhee, P.E. (Ed.). (1989). *Humor and children's development: A guide to practical applications.* New York: Haworth Press.

McGhee, P.E. (1994). *How to develop your sense of humor: An 8-step humor development training program for learning to use humor to cope with stress.* Dubuque, IA: Kendall/Hunt Publishing.

McGhee, P.E. (2000). Humor and laughter strengthen your immune system. In P.E. McGhee, *Health, healing and the amuse system: Humor as survival training.* [Electronic Resource]. Retrieved February 18, 2009, from http://www.humor.ch/mcghee/mcghee_00_01. htm

McGhee, P.E. (2001). *Humor your tumor.* Retrieved February 18, 2009, from http://www .laughterremedy.com/humor2.dir/humor 5_01.html

McMahan, S.C. (2008). Infinite possibility: Clowning with elderly people. *Care Management Journals, 9*(1), 19-24.

Merriam, S.B. & Brockett, R.G. (1997). *The profession and practice of adult education: An introduction.* San Francisco: Jossey-Bass.

Millbower, L (2010). Humor Project puts the laughs in learning at its upcoming conference - part two. Retrieved June 10, 2010, from http://www.examiner.com/x-8694-Presentation-Skills-Examiner~y2010m2d18-Humor-Project-puts-the-laughs-in-learning-at-its-upcoming-conference--part-two

Minden, P. (2002). Humor as the focal point of treatment for forensic psychiatric patients. *Holistic Nursing Practice, 16*(4), 75-86.

Moore, S. (2002). *Math quiz for emergency department staff.* Retrieved February 18, 2009, from http://www.joke-archives.com/medical/math quizfortheemergencydeptstaff.html

Moss, S.W. (2004). Marriage enhancement through humor. Doctorial Dissertation. Union Institute & University. UMI Number 3251488. Retrieved November 26, 2008, from UMI ProQuest Digital Dissertations.

Murphy, J.R. (1978). Is it Skinner or nothing? In M. Knowles (Ed.), *Adult learner: A neglected species,* Vol. 2. Houston: Gulf.

Newirth, J. (2006) The analyst as comic and the comic in analysis: Reply to commentary. *Psychoanalytic Dialogues, 16*(5), 579-584.

Newman, B.M. & Newman, P.R. (1999). *Development through life: A psychological approach* (7th ed). Pacific Grove: Brooks/Cole.

Nezu, A.M., Nezu, C.M., & Blissett, S.E. (1988) Sense of humor as a moderator of the relation between stressful events and psychological distress: A prospective analysis. *Journal of Personality and Social Psychology, 54*(3), 520-525.

Our ancient laughing brain. (n.d.) *Mind and behavior.* Retrieved November 3, 2008 from http://www.cerebromente.org.br/n13/mente/laughter/page5.html

Pajares, F. (1997, July 7). *Overview of social cognitive theory.* Retrieved March 1, 2009, from http://www.emory.edu/EDUCATION/mfp/eff.html

Pasquali, E.A. (1990). Learning to laugh: Humor as therapy. *Journal of Psychosocial Nursing and Mental Health Services, 28*(3), 31-35.

Pasquali, E.A. (1995). Humor for mentally ill patients. In K. Buxman & A. LeMoine (Eds.), *Nursing perspectives on humor.* Staten Island, NY: Power Publications.

Peterson, K. (2007). Humor in children: A potential buffer again rejection and depression in first-grade children. Doctorial Dissertation. Seattle Pacific University. UMI Number: 3267401. Retrieved May 15, 2008, from UMI ProQuest Digital Dissertations.

Petzall, K. & Olsson H. (2007). Subjective well-being in old age: a Swedish interventional study. *Nursing Science & Research in the Nordic Countries, 27*(4), 9.

Porterfield, A. (1987). Does sense of humor moderate the impact of life stress on psychological and physical well-being? *Journal of Research in Personality, 21,* 306-317.

Prerost, F.J. (n.d.) Children and humor: Parent handout. National Association Of School Psychologists. Retrieved March 15, 2009, from http://www.amphi.com/~psych/humor.html

Provine, R.R. (2000a). *Laughter: A scientific investigation.* New York: Viking.

Provine, R.R. (2000b). The science of laughter. *Psychology Today, 33*(6), 58-61. Retrieved July 3, 2003, from EBSCO Host database.

Provine, R. (2004, December). Laughing, Tickling, and the Evolution of Speech and Self. *Current Directions in Psychological Science, 13,* 215-218.

Reddy, V., Williams, E., & Vaughan, A. (2002). Sharing laughter: The humour of pre-school children with *Down syndrome. Down's Syndrome Research and Practice, 7*(3), 125-128.

Ritz, S.E. (1995). Survivor humor and disaster nursing. In K. Buxman & A. LeMoine (Eds.), *Nursing perspectives on humor.* Staten Island, NY: Power Publications.

Robinson, D.T. & Smith-Lovin, L. (2001). Getting a laugh: Gender, status, and humor in task discussions. *Social Forces, 80*(1), 123-158.

Robinson, V. (1978) *Humor and the health professions* (1st ed). Thorofare, NJ: Slack.

Robinson, V.M. (1991) *Humor and the health professions* (2nd ed). Thorofare, NJ: Slack.

Robinson, V.M. (1995). Humor in nursing: A hysterical perspective. In K. Buxman & A. LeMoine (Eds), *Nursing perspectives on humor (pp. 9-17)*. Staten Island, NY: Power Publications.

Rosner, F. (2002). Therapeutic efficacy of laughter in medicine. *Cancer Investigation, 20*(3) 434-436.

Rupert, P.A. & Kent, J.S. (2007. Gender and work setting differences in career-sustaining behaviors and burnout among professional psychologists. *Professional Psychology: Research and Practice, 38*(1), 88-96.

Ruch, W., McGhee, P.E., & Hehl, F.J. (1990). Age differences in the enjoyment of incongruity-resolution and nonsense humor during adulthood. *Psychology and Aging, 5*(3), 348-355.

Rx Laughter. (2002). *Laughter tested as pain therapy for children*. Retrieved February 18, 2009, from http://www.rxlaughter.org/pAMA.htm

Sakowicz, E. (2007). *Laughter is cheap medicine.* Retrieved November 19, 2008, from http://www.ikidney.com/article.php?id=2007 0208010815

Sahaklan, A & Frishman, W.H. (2007). Humor and the cardiovascular system. *Alternative Therapies in Health and Medicine, 13*(4), 56-58.

Salameh, W.A. (1983). Humor in psychotherapy: Past outlooks, present status, and future frontiers. In P.E. McGhee & J.H. Goldstein (Eds.), *Handbook of humor research: Vol. II* (pp. 61-85). New York: Springer-Verlag.

Schleifer, S.J., Keller, S.E., Bartlett, J.A., Eckholdt, H.M., & Delaney, B.R. (1996). Immunity in young adults with major depressive disorder. *American Journal of Psychiatry, 153*(4), 477-482.

Schrecengost, A. (2001). Do humorous preoperative teaching strategies work? *AORN Journal, 74*(5), 683-689.

Schunk, D.H. (1991). *Learning theories: An educational perspective.* New York: Merrill.

Schwartz, E.A. (2006). The use of humor in coping with breast cancer. Doctoral Dissertation, Walden University. (Publication Number: AAT 3244620). Retrieved May 8, 2008, from UMI ProQuest Digital Dissertations.

Schwebke, S. (n.d.). *The hospital clown: A closer look.* Retrieved February 18, 2009, from http://www.hospitalclown.com

Schwebke, S. (n.d.). I love you Wollie. *The Hospital Clown Newsletter.* Retrieved February 18, 2009, from http://www.hospitalclown.com/ InfoPages/storiesTable.htm

Seaward, B.L. (1992, April). Humor's healing potential. *Health Progress, 73*(3), 66-70.

Shade, R. (1991). Verbal humor in gifted students and students in the general population: A comparison of spontaneous mirth and comprehension. *Journal for the Education of the Gifted, 14*(2), 134-150.

Shelley, C. (2003). "Plato on the psychology of humor," *HUMOR: International Journal of humor research 16*(4), 351–368.

Shibles, W. (2002). *Humor reference guide: A comprehensive classification and analysis.* Retrieved January 25, 2009, from http:// www.drbarbaramaier.at/shiblesw

Smitt, M. (1995, November). *Humor and hospice...Not an oxymoron.* Handout from the annual meeting of the American Association of Therapeutic Humor.

Socha, T.J. (1994). Children making "fun:" Humorous communication, impression management, and moral development. *Child Study Journal, 24*(3), 237-253.

Solomon, J.C. (1996, January). Humor and aging well: A laughing matter or a matter of laughing. *American Behavioral Scientist, 39*(3), 249-272.

Stanhope, M. & Lancaster J. (2004). *Community and public health nursing,* 6th ed. St. Louis: Mosby.

Stewart, C. (2008) *Mental health humor and cartoons.* Retrieved Dec. 1, 2008, from http://mental healthhumor.today.com

Strubbe, B. (2003). Getting serious about laughter. *The World and I, 18*(3), 132-140. Retrieved May 29, 2003, from EBSCO Host database.

Struthers, J. (1999). An investigation into community psychiatric nurses' use of humour during client interactions. *Journal of Advanced Nursing, 29*(5), 1197-1204.

Stuart, G.W. & Sundeen, S.J. (Eds.) (1995). *Principles and practice of psychiatric nursing* (5th ed.). St. Louis: Mosby.

Stuber, M., Dunay Hilber, S., Libman Mintzer, L., Castaneda, M., Glover, D., & Zeltzer, L. (2009). Laughter, Humor and Pain Perception in Children: A Pilot Study. *eCAM. 6*(2), 271–276.

Sultanoff, S.M. (1992). *The impact of humor in the counseling relationship.* Originally published in *Laugh it Up.* Retrieved March 3, 2009, from http://www.humormatters.com/articles/therapy 2.htm

Sultanoff, S.M. (1994). Choosing the amusing: Assessing the individual's receptivity to therapeutic humor. *Journal of Nursing Jocularity 4*(4), 35-35.

Sultanoff, S.M. (1995). *Levity defies gravity: Using humor in crisis situations.* Retrieved February 18, 2009, from Association for Applied and Therapeutic Humor at http://www.aath.org/articles/art_sultanoff02.html

Sultanoff, S.M. (2000). Using humor for treatment and diagnosis: A shrinking perspective. Originally published in *Therapeutic Humor, 15*(1), 5. Retrieved February 18, 2009, from http://www.humormatters.com/articles/treatmentdiagnosis.htm

Sultanoff, S.M. (2009). *Revisiting the land of mirth and funny.* Retrieved May 9, 2009 from http://www.journalofnursingjocularity.com/2009/04/13/rivisiting-the-land-of-mirth-and-funny-by-steve-sultanoff-phd/#more-1747

Tan, S.A., Tan, L.G., Berk, L.S., Lukman, S.T., & Lukman, L.F. (1997). Mirthful laughter, an effective adjunct in cardiac rehabilitation. *Canadian Journal of Cardiology, 13*(suppl B), 190.

Taylor, I. & Burgess, H. (1995). Orientation to self directed learning. Paradox or paradigm. *Studies in Higher Education, 20*(1). Retrieved March 4, 2009, from EBSCO Host database.

Thompson-Richards, J. (2006) Joy in the midst of suffering: Clowning as care of the spirit in palliative care. *Aging, Spirituality, and Palliative Care, 18*(2/3), 137-152.

Tumkaya, S. (2007) Burnout and humor relationship among university lecturers. *Humor: International Journal of Humor Research,* (20)1, 73-92.

Uekermann, J., Daum, I, & Channon, S. (2007). Toward a cognitive and social neuroscience of humor processing. *Social Cognition, 25*(4), 553-572.

University of Maryland Medical Center (2005, March 16). *Laughter helps blood vessels function better.* Retrieved March 9, 2009, from www.sciencedaily.com/releases/2005/03/050309111444.htm

Vella, J. (1994). Learning to listen/learning to teach: Training trainers in the principles and practices of popular education. *Convergence, 27*(1).

Wade, S.L., Borawski, E.A., Taylor, H.G., Drotar, D., Yeates, K.O., & Stancin, T. (2001). The relationship of caregiver coping to family outcomes during the initial year following pediatric traumatic injury. *Journal of Consulting and Clinical Psychology, 69*(3), 406-415.

Walsh, T. (n.d.). Funny heart protection: Laughing makes the heart grow stronger. *Healthy Heart Center.* Retrieved March 10, 2009, from http://www.prevention.com/cda/article/funny heart-protection/026166263d803110VgnVCM 20000012281eac_/health/emotional.health

Warren, J.E., Sauter, D.A., Eisner, F., Wiland, J., Dresner, A., Wise, R.J.S., et al. (2006). Positive emotions preferentially engage an ausitory-motor "mirror" system. *The Journal of Neuroscience, 26*(50), 13067-13075.

Watkins, A. (1997). Mind-body pathways. In A. Watkins (Ed.), *Mind-Body Medicine.* New York: Churchill Livingstone.

Watson, A. (2001). Sadie, Sadie, special lady. In J. Canfield, M.V. Hansen, N. Mitchell-Autio, & L. Thieman (Eds.), *Chicken Soup for the Nurse's Soul.* Deerfield Beach, FL: Health Communications, Inc.

Webster's New World College Dictionary. (2010). Cleveland, OH: Wiley Publishing, Inc.

Weeks, L. (02/27/2006). The Nawlins muck, Thery're yucking it up. *The Washington Post.* Retrieved November 8, 2009, from Ebscohost.

Wells, K. (2001). Humor therapy. In K.M. Krapp & J.L. Longe (Eds.), *The Gale Encyclopedia of Alternative Medicine.* Detroit, MI: Thomson Gale.

Whisonant, R.D. (1998). *The effects of humor on cognitive learning in a computer-based environment.* Doctorial Dissertation, Virginia Polytechnic Institute. (Publication Number: AAT 9905176). Retrieved March 8, 2005, from UMI ProQuest Digital Dissertations.

Wilson, C.P. (1979). *Jokes: Form, content, use, and function.* New York: Academic Press.

Wiklinski, B.A. (1994). Has humor a meaning for persons adapting to a cancer experience? A phenomenological question (UMI No. 75009). *Dissertation Abstracts International: Section B: The Sciences & Engineering, 54*(12-B).

Wlodkowski, R.J. (1990). Strategies to enhance adult motivation to learn. In M.W. Galbraith (Ed.), *Adult learning methods: A guide for effective instruction.* Malabar, FL: R.E. Krieger.

Wong, P.T. (2003). Humor and laughter in wartime. *International Network on Personal Meaning.* Retrieved March 3, 2009, from http://www.meaning.ca/archives/pres_cols.html

Wooten, P. (1992). Send in the clowns! Part I. *Journal of Nursing Jocularity, 2*(4), 46-47.

Wooten, P. (1994). *Jest for the health of it!: An interview with William Fry, Jr., MD.*

Wooten, P. (1995). Humor cart for cancer patients: Interview with Terry Bennett. *Journal of Nursing Jocularity, 5*(3), 46-47.

Wooten, P. (1996). Humor: An antidote for stress. *Holistic Nursing Practice, 10*(2), 49-55. Retrieved May 28, 2003, from http://www.jest health.com/images/HumorStressAntidote.pdf

Wooten, P. (1997). You've got to be kidding! Humor skills for surviving managed care. *Dermatology Nursing, 9*(6), pp. 423-428.

Wooten, P. & Dunkelblau, E. (2001). *Tragedy, laughter, and survival.* Retrieved May 24, 2003, from, http://www.aath.org/art_wootdunk1.html

World Laughter Tour. (n.d.). *Our History.* Retrieved July 1, 2003, from http://www.worldlaughtertour.com/sections/about/history.asp

Yale–New Haven Children's Hospital. (2002). *Big Apple Circus Clown Care Unit.* Retrieved March 10, 2009, from http://www.ynhh.org/pediatrics/support/clown_care_unit.html

Zemke, R. &. Zemke, S. (1984, March 9). 30 things we know for sure about adult learning. *Innovative Abstracts VI*(8). National Institute for Staff and Organizational Development. Retrieved March 10, 2009, from http://honolulu.hawaii.edu/intranet/committees/FacDevCom/guidebk/teachtip/adults-3.htm

Ziegler, J.B. (1998). Use of humor in medical teaching. *Medical Teacher, 20*(4), 341-348.

Ziv, A. (1984). *Personality and sense of humor.* New York: Springer Publishing.

INDEX